Immunology for Pharmacy Students

Other books of interest

Basic Endocrinology – For Students of Pharmacy and Allied Health Sciences
A. Constanti and A. Bartke with clinical case studies by R. Khardori

Pharmaceutical Biotechnology – An Introduction for Pharmacists and Pharmaceutical Scientists
D.J.A. Crommelin and R.D. Sindelar

Forthcoming

Drug Delivery and Targeting – For Pharmacists and Pharmaceutical Scientists
A.M. Hillery, A.W. Lloyd and J. Swarbrick

Immunology for Pharmacy Students

Wei-Chiang Shen
and
Stan G. Louie
School of Pharmacy, University of Southern California, Los Angeles, USA

ho **harwood academic publishers**
ap Australia • Canada • China • France • Germany • India • Japan • Luxembourg
Malaysia • The Netherlands • Russia • Singapore • Switzerland

Amsteldijk 166
1st Floor
1079 LH Amsterdam
The Netherlands

British Library Cataloguing in Publication Data

A catalogue record for this book is available from the British Library.

ISBN: 90-5702-380-6 (softcover)

Table of Contents

Chapter 10: **Immunodiagnostics and Immunoassays**   *131*

Appendices: **Immunological Agents as Therapeutic Drugs**   *149*

Preface

Modern immunology evolved almost a century ago with the discovery of vaccines and antitoxins. Therefore, the development of pharmaceutical agents for the treatment or prevention of human diseases was a major driving force behind the establishment of immunology as a scientific discipline. As the field of immunology flourished and matured into a basic science discipline, less attention was focused on the therapeutic aspects. This was primarily due to the inability to produce sufficient amounts of immune factors or components for clinical use.

However, major advances in biotechnology have allowed the mass production of immune-derived factors and antibodies, enabling production of large quantities for both basic and clinical uses. Immunotherapy and immunodiagnostics have impacted the way patients are managed, thus necessitating prompt interfacing of basic science with clinical applications. The ability to produce large amounts of immune factors has also enabled researchers to probe the various activities of the immune system, and to examine how these newly discovered immune factors can be used as pharmaceutical agents. This textbook highlights such advances in basic science and also in more applied clinical issues.

Given the large number of recombinant pharmaceutical and diagnostic agents that have entered the clinical arena, it is not surprising that an increasing number of pharmacy schools have added immunology to their curriculum.

Despite this rapid movement towards incorporation of immunology into pharmacy education, there are relatively few books that address the issues that are germane to pharmacy students. Most textbooks are either unable to be incorporated into the intensive pharmacy curriculum, or lack the depth and discussion of issues that are essential for pharmacists such as drug allergies, antibody therapy, immunotherapy, and vaccines.

This book was written based on our experience in teaching immunology to pharmacy students during the last several years at the University of Southern California (USC). It is intended to be used for a two- to three-unit course in one semester, as the immunology course is currently offered in most pharmacy schools. We would like to thank the many pharmacy students at USC, who have provided us with valuable feedback in our lectures during these years. Their input has helped to shape the content of this textbook. We would also like to thank the following graduate students in the laboratory of Wei-Chiang Shen: Mitchell Taub, Laura Honeycutt, and Karin Boulossow, for their comments and suggestions on the manuscript of this book. Finally, special acknowledgments are given to Jerry Shen for his work on the figures in this book, and to Cornelia Hatten for her patience and assistance in preparing the manuscript.

Wei-Chiang Shen and **Stan G. Louie**

Acknowledgements

The cover illustration and all figures were designed by Jerry Shen.

I Introduction

Immunology and Pharmaceutics

Immunology is a discipline in the biomedical sciences dealing with the mechanisms and structures in a living organism (including man) for protection against infectious diseases. The evolution of living organisms on earth has resulted in the development of various self-defense systems to prevent the proliferation of microorganisms such as bacteria, fungi, protozoa, and viruses which constantly search for hosts to infect. Without this immunity, it would be impossible for higher organisms to exist on earth. The self-defense system has evolved into a complicated infrastructure (immune system) in vertebrates, which not only acts to prevent infections but occasionally can cause various diseases itself (immunopathology).

Knowledge of immunology is important for pharmacy practice and pharmaceutical research (Figure 1.1). Drugs affecting the immune system can be used for the treatment of immunological diseases such as allergies, immune deficiencies, and transplantation (Chapters 5, 6 and 8). On the other hand, immunological factors such as antibodies and cytokines, which can be isolated from the blood or produced by biotechnological methods, can be used as drugs for the treatment of various diseases including cancer and AIDS (Chapters 4, and 7). In addition, antibodies can be used as analytical reagents for diagnostic and drug screening applications when a highly specific and sensitive assay procedure is required (Chapter 10). Finally, knowledge of immunology also is important for the understanding and the treatment of allergic reactions to drugs (Chapter 5).

Organs and Cells in the Immune System

Bone marrow, the thymus gland, spleen, and lymph nodes are organs that are necessary for the normal functioning of the human immune system. These organs are connected by a network of lymphatic vessels in which lymphatic fluid moves from organ to organ in a fashion analogous to the circulation of blood in the vascular network. However, unlike the blood, lymphatic fluid is devoid of erythrocytes, being only enriched with leukocytes. The lymphatic network plays an important role in the body's response to local infections. In addition, lymphatic vessels are also involved in the elimination of exogenous macromolecules from tissues, which may have implications for the clearance of macromolecules or polymers from the target sites in macromolecule-mediated drug delivery.

The immune system in vertebrates can best be described in terms of its constituent cells. As shown in Figure 1.2,

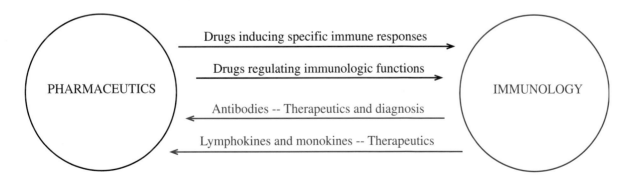

Figure 1.1. The interrelationship between pharmaceutics and immunology. Drugs such as immunosuppressors, immunomodulators, and vaccines are important tools for the study of immunology as well as the treatment of immunological disorders. On the other hand, immunological components such as antibodies and interleukins are becoming increasingly important as drugs produced by pharmaceutical industries for the treatment of various diseases, including cancer and AIDS.

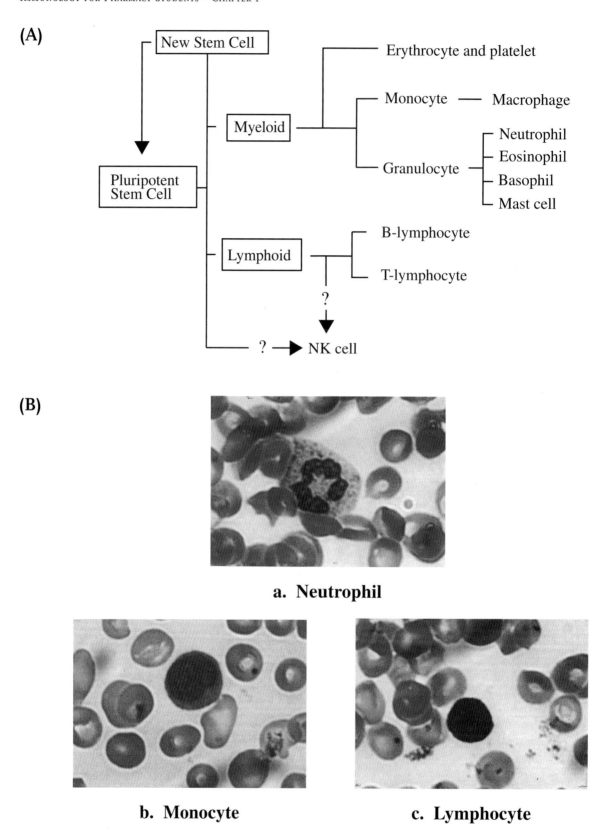

a. Neutrophil

b. Monocyte　　　　**c. Lymphocyte**

Figure 1.2. (A) Cells in the immune system. All cells in the immune system are derived from pluripotent stem cells. Stem cells differentiate into two major cell lineages, i.e., myeloid and lymphoid. It is uncertain whether natural killer (NK) cells are derived from lymphoid cells or from a third lineage. Pluripotent stem cells also proliferate to generate new stem cells. (B) Three most commonly found leukocytes in human blood. (a) a neutrophil, (b) a monocyte and (c) a lymphocyte.

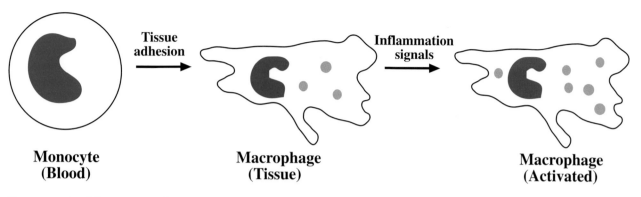

Figure 1.3. The differentiation of a monocyte to a macrophage. Monocytes in the blood have a relatively short half-life, i.e., less than 10 hr, before they become tissue-associated. Once in the tissue, monocytes differentiate into various types of macrophages with the morphology and function largely dependent on the environment of the tissue that they reside in. Upon being challenged by inflammatory signals such as complement factors and cytokines, macrophages can be activated and become highly phagocytic with increasing number and size of granules in the cytoplasm.

cells which participate in the adult human immune system all originate from pluripotent stem cells residing in the bone marrow. Stem cells can differentiate into two different lineages of cells, i.e., myeloid and lymphoid cells. Many important blood cells such as erythrocytes and platelets are derived from myeloid cells, as are many leukocytes. There are two classes of leukocytes which belong to the myeloid lineage: the granulocytes or polymorphonuclear leukocytes (PMN), named after the multi-lobed morphology of their nuclei and the presence of multiple granules in their cytoplasm. There are three major types of granulocytes in the blood: neutrophils, eosinophils, and basophils. Neutrophils are the most predominant leukocytes, representing approximately 50–75% of blood leukocytes (Figure 1.2). Their size (9–10 µm) is larger than that of erythrocytes (7 µm), but their life in the blood circulation after leaving the bone marrow is less than 10 hours. The cytoplasm of a neutrophil contains many weakly stained granules, which are the lysosomes and phagosomes. Eosinophils comprise only 2–4% of blood leukocytes. Their cytoplasm contains many granules which can be intensively stained using eosin dye. These granules are packed with many inflammatory mediators such as leukotrienes which are released when the cell comes in contact with infectious microorganisms, particularly parasites. Basophils comprise only less than 0.2% of blood leukocytes. Their cytoplasmic granules contain heparin and histamine which are powerful anticoagulant and vasoactive agents. Their specific role in the immune response is not clear; however, like eosinophils, basophils may be important in the immune response against parasites. Mast cells, which are best known for their involvement in allergic reactions (Chapter 7), are similar to basophils except that they are associated with mucosal and connective tissues rather than with the blood. The other type of blood leukocyte is the monocyte. Monocytes differ from granulocytes in their size (12–15 µm), nuclear morphology

(horse-shoe shape), and plasma membrane markers (Figure 1.2). Monocytes have a short half-life of less than 10 hours in the blood circulation before they migrate and attach to various tissues and differentiate into macrophages. Therefore, macrophages are terminally differentiated, tissue-associated monocytes (Figure 1.3). Macrophages are large (15–20 µm) and express a high phagocytic activity. Most importantly, unlike granulocytes which are only cytodestructive leukocytes, monocytes and macrophages are also responsible for the recognition and presentation of antigens in the acquired immune response (Chapters 2 and 3). Furthermore, monocytes and macrophages are sources of many secretory factors (e.g., complements and monokines) which are also important factors governing the acquired immune response.

The lymphoid cells differentiate into two types of lymphocytes, i.e., T-lymphocytes and B-lymphocytes, which represent 20–45% of blood leukocytes with a size which is only slightly larger than that of an erythrocyte. However, lymphocytes have a very large nucleus which makes them distinguishable from enucleated erythrocytes (Figure 1.2). T-lymphocytes are the major cells involved in the cellular immunity (Chapter 3), while B-lymphocytes are the cells which can further differentiate into antibody-producing plasma cells in humoral immunity (Chapter 2). T and B cells can be distinguished from each other by their membrane associated markers; the most apparent difference is that B-lymphocytes express immunoglobulin molecules (antibodies) on their membrane and T-lymphocytes express different T cell receptors such as CD3 and CD4 or CD8 (Chapter 3). Both T- and B-lymphocytes are originally differentiated from stem cells in the bone marrow. B-lymphocytes mature in the bone marrow before they migrate into the blood and other lymphatic tissues such as lymph nodes and the spleen. T-lymphocytes, on the other hand, leave the bone marrow as thymocytes and migrate to the thymus. It is in the thymic gland that a small fraction of thymocytes further differentiate into mature T-lymphocytes which migrate from the thymic gland to the blood and other lymphatic tissues.

There are other minor types of cells in the immune system such as the natural killer (NK) cells which may be either derived from lymphoid cells, as named large granular lymphocytes (LGL), or from a third lineage in the differentiation of the stem cells.

Divisions of the Immune System

Immunity in vertebrates can be divided into different sections. By the processes involved in the immune response, an immune system consists of innate immunity and acquired immunity. By the components involved in the immune response, an immune system can be divided into humoral immunity and cellular immunity. Finally, by the location of the immune response, an immune system consists of serosal immunity and mucosal immunity. These different forms of immunity will be described within several chapters in this book. In this chapter, we will review first the innate immunity — the most basic form of defense against infections in vertebrates.

Innate Immunity

Innate immunity includes immune mechanisms which are present constantly in the organism from birth. Innate immunity is different from acquired immunity which is also called adaptive immunity. Innate immunity is the first line of defense mechanisms against infections; it is a fast response, non-specific, and does not have a memory with respect to previous infections. On the other hand, acquired immunity is developed only after the invasion of an infectious agent; it is slow in response to infection, highly specific, and, most importantly, can have a memory of previous infections so that it will have a fast response when the infection recurs (Figure 1.4).

Innate immunity consists of three different components: physical barriers, cells, and soluble factors. The physical barriers include the skin, mucosa, and mucus. Skin provides the most important physical protection of the body against hazardous conditions, including physical, chemical, and biological insults from the environment. Protection by the skin is primarily due to the existence of the stratum corneum which is a keratinized layer of protein and lipid. On mucosal surfaces such as the nasal and gastrointestinal surfaces, protection is provided by epithelium. An epithelium consists of a monolayer or multilayer of epithelial cells with tight-junctions between adjacent cells to provide an impermeable physical barrier, thus keeping

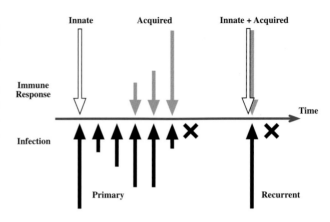

Figure 1.4. The involvement of innate and acquired immunity against infection. When encountering a primary challenge (black arrow), the immediate response of the immune system is via the innate immunity (white arrow). The innate immunity is quick but nonspecific to the infectious agents, and therefore, is less effective. However, the innate immunity can slow down the infection significantly and during this period of time the acquired immunity (blue arrow) can be developed. The acquired immunity is highly selective to the specific infectious agent and can completely stop the infection process (black cross). In the future, if the same infection recurs, the acquired immunity can respond immediately together with the innate immunity to ensure a rapid elimination of the infection.

microorganisms out of the body. In most epithelia, further protection is provided by the secretion of mucus from special types of epithelial cells such as goblet cells in gastrointestinal mucosa. Mucus is a viscous liquid layer mostly consisting of an acidic glycoprotein, mucin. Mucus can render macromolecules and microorganisms inaccessible to the membrane of epithelial cells; thus, the possibility of infection by various pathogens can be significantly decreased. When the skin or the epithelium is injured, an infection is almost inevitable and other innate immune components will then be needed to respond the challenge.

The cellular components of the innate immune response include granulocytes in the blood and macrophages in the tissues. The major granulocyte in the blood is the neutrophils. When infection by a microorganism occurs in the tissue, chemotactic factors will be generated at the infectious site which can make the capillary blood vessel endothelium leaky; neutrophils will then be attracted to cross the capillary endothelium (Figure 1.5). There are three types of chemotactic factors: (1) formylmethionyl peptides generated from bacteria, (2) factors secreted by phagocytes such as leukotrienes, and (3) peptide fragments from activated complement proteins such as C3a and C5a. Neutrophils and macrophages are capable of engulfing and destroying

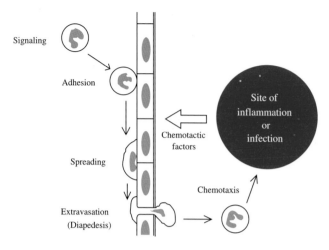

Tissue	Cell
Liver	Kupffer cells
Lung	Alveolar macrophages
Peritoneum	Peritoneal macrophages
Spleen	Dendritic cells
Skin	Langerhans cells
Brain	Microglial cells

Table 1.1. Cells in the reticuloendothelial system.

Figure 1.5. The process of chemotaxis. Endothelial cells respond to the chemotactic and inflammatory factors generated at the site of inflammation or infection by releasing mediators which serve as signals to attract blood granulocytes and by expressing adhesive proteins on the surface to bind those attracted granulocytes. After adhesion and spreading on the endothelial surface, granulocytes migrate across the blood vessel through the endothelial cell gaps to reach the site of inflammation or infection; a process called "diapedesis." Many proteins are involved in this process, such as selectins and intercellular adhesive molecules (ICAM-1) on the surface of endothelial cells to bind integrins on the surface of granulocytes. Vasodilators, such as tumor-necrosis factor (TNF-α) and leukotrienes, are involved in loosening the cell–cell gap junction. TNF-α is also involved in the induction of adhesive proteins on the surface of endothelial cells.

microorganisms by a process called phagocytosis (Figure 1.6); they are called phagocytes, or phagocytic cells. Non-phagocytic cells are also involved in innate immunity. These types of cell, which can kill target cells by releasing cytotoxic factors, are called cytotoxic cells. Basophils, eosinophils, and NK cells are cytotoxic cells involved in the innate immune response. As will be described in the later chapters, phagocytic cells such as macrophages and cytotoxic cells such as cytotoxic T-cells are also involved in the acquired immunity. In tissues, the major type of cells involved in innate immunity are the macrophages. Tissue macrophages differentiate from circulated monocytes in the blood. Monocytes differentiate into various types of macrophages such as Kupffer's cells in the liver and aveolar macrophages in the lungs; this differentiation depends upon the tissue in which they reside (Table 1.1). The tissue-associated macrophage network is referred to as the reticuloendothelial system (RES).

Individuals with a defect in either the number or the activity of phagocytes are deficient in this self-defense sys-

tem, and consequently are vulnerable to many infectious diseases. This immune deficient condition can be a result of many different causes. Genetic deficiencies of enzymes such as myeloperoxidase and glucose-6-phosphate dehydrogenase can decrease the activity of phagocytes in the ingestion and killing of bacteria. A deficiency in the production of chemotactic factors can also decrease the activity of phagocytes. Genetic disorder in phagocytic activity is found to be the cause of chronic granulomatous disease (CGD), in which macrophages with accumulated particles in large granules in the cytoplasm are found to fuse with each other as a result of the inability to break down ingested materials. Another type of phagocytosis deficiency, leukopenia, is due to the low number of phagocytes in the blood. Depending on the type of deficient leukocyte, this disorder can also be called neutropenia or granulocytopenia. Leukopenia can be due to a genetic deficiency in producing mature leukocytes; it can also be caused by environmental factors such as overexposure to radiation or an overdose of certain cancer chemotherapeutic drugs having bone marrow toxicity. Because of the short life of granulocytes in circulation, the transfusion of blood cells is not a very effective treatment for leukopenia. On the other hand, bone marrow transplantation can be used as an alternative treatment, but certain risks and complications of this treatment must be considered (Chapter 8). Recently, recombinant colony-stimulating factors for granulocytes and macrophages (G-CSF and GM-CSF, Chapter 2 and 7) have become commercially available for therapeutic applications; these factors provide a new approach for the treatment of these diseases. In addition to self defense, neutrophils and macrophages are responsible for many pathological inflammatory conditions, e.g., rheumatoid arthritis and asthma attacks. Therefore, agents that can interfere with the activity of phagocytes are currently being tested as drugs for the treatment of these disorders.

Soluble factors in the innate immunity consist of: (1) bactericidal factors, (2) complements, and (3) interferons.

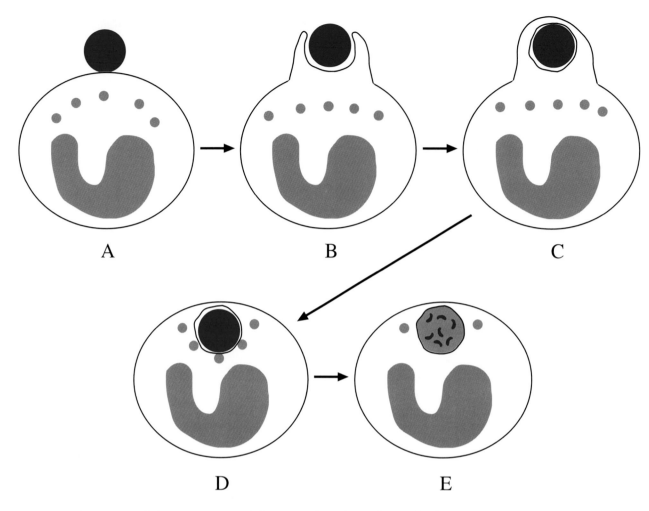

Figure 1.6. The process of phagocytosis. (A) A foreign particle such as a bacterial cell is attached to the membrane of a phagocyte via specific or nonspecific interactions. (B) The multiple interaction between the surfaces of the particle and the phagocyte induces the formation of pseudopods around the particle. (C) The fusion of the pseudopods includes the particle to form a phagosome in the cytoplasm of the phagocyte. (D) The phagosome migrates towards the perinuclear region of the phagocyte and fuses with lysosomes to become a phagolysosome. (E) Inside the phagolysosome, the particle is digested by lysosomal enzymes.

Bactericidal Factors

The most primitive bactericidal factor in the human body is hydrochloric acid which is secreted by the parietal cells of the stomach epithelial lining. Besides activating pepsin and promoting the hydrolysis of food, the extremely acidic condition in the stomach also kills many bacteria and other microorganisms that are taken up orally. Other bactericidal factors are generally produced by either phagocytes or hepatocytes. Phagocytes release many factors, most of them directed to the phagosomes in order to kill the ingested microorganisms (Table 1.2). The most important mechanism in this phagocytic killing are superoxide and hydrogen peroxide production, a process referred to as the respiratory burst. Failure to generate the respiratory burst due to

Factor	Formation	Site of action
Oxygen ions and radicals	Induced	Phagosomes
Acid hydrolases	Preformed	Lysosomes
Cationic proteins	Preformed	Phagosomes
Defensins	Preformed	Phagosomes or extracellular
Lactoferrin, etc.	Preformed	Phagosomes

Table 1.2. Antimicrobial factors produced by phagocytes.

a genetic deficiency in the oxidase enzyme is the major cause of the chronic granulomatous disease. In addition to the respiratory burst, there are many other antimicrobial factors which are released from phagocytes. Among these factors are defensins, formerly known lysosomal cationic proteins. Defensins are a group of arginine and cystine-rich antimicrobial peptides having 29 to 35 amino acid residues and constituting more than 5% of the total cellular proteins in human neutrophils. Defensins have a very broad antimicrobial spectrum including activity against both gram-positive and gram-negative bacteria, fungi, and certain types of viruses. The exact mechanism of defensins on the killing of microorganisms is still unknown; however, it has been suggested that defensins can exert their antimicrobial activity by the electrostatic interaction with negatively charged surface molecules and subsequently altering the membrane permeability of the target cells. Another important bactericidal factor released from phagocytes is lysozyme. Lysozyme is a cationic protein of 14 kDa molecular weight with an enzymatic activity which hydrolyzes the beta 1–4 glycosidic linkage of the polysaccharides in the bacterial cell wall. The hydrolysis of this bacterial cell wall-specific polysaccharide will cause bacterial lysis. Lysozyme has been detected in almost all of physiological fluids, including saliva and tears. During inflammation or infection, the release of hepatocyte-produced proteins into the serum may occur. These proteins are generally called acute phase proteins (Table 1.3). Most acute phase proteins do not act directly on bacteria,

Factor	Activity
C-reactive protein (CRP)	Chemotaxis and phagocytosis enhancement
α_1-antitrypsin	Protease inhibition
Fibrinogen	Coagulation
Complement factors	Complement activation

Table 1.3. Acute phase proteins.

but rather enhance the bactericidal activity of other factors or cells.

Complement Pathways

One of the major serum components for defense against bacterial infection is the complement system. Complements are a group of glycoproteins which can be activated during the acquired immune response to induce antibody-mediated cytotoxicity (Chapter 3). However, the complement system can act directly on the surface of bacteria without the involvement of antibodies. This activation mechanism is called the alternative pathway so as to distinguish it from the classical pathway of acquired immunity (Figure 1.7).

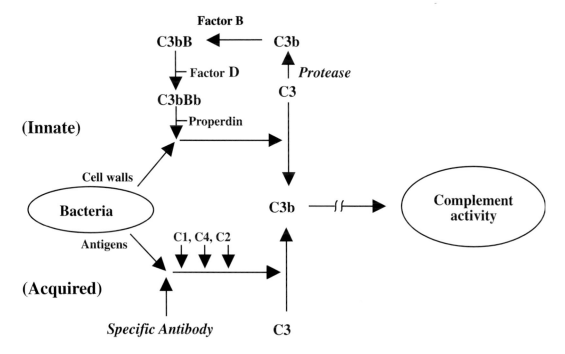

Figure 1.7. Comparison of the alternative (innate) and the classical (acquired) complement pathways. The innate pathway is initiated by the proteolytic conversion of C3 to C3b and the formation of C3bBb complexes in the blood which subsequently will bind polysaccharides on the bacterial cell walls. The acquired pathway is initiated by the recognition of specific antibodies against antigens on the surface of target cells. Details of the pathways will be discussed in Chapter 3: Antibodies and Complements.

	Type I		Type II
	IFN-α	IFN-β	IFN-γ
Producing cells	Leukocytes	Fibroblasts	T-lymphocytes
Producing mechanism		Viral infection	Mitogen-stimulation
Isotypes	17	1	1
Molecular weight (kDa)	16–27	20	20–24
Receptor	Identical (95–110 kDa)		90–95 kDa

Table 1.4. Human interferons.

The alternative pathway is initiated by a small amount of complement factor C3 in the serum which is converted by serum proteases to a C3b fragment. C3b in the serum binds to another complement factor B and the C3bB complex is subsequently converted by factor D in the serum to C3bBb by breaking down B into Bb. C3bBb binds with another serum factor, properdin, to give PC3bBb complex which in turn binds to polysaccharide components in the bacterial cell wall. The binding of PC3bBb complex will initiate a cascade of complement factor activation, involving factors from C5 to C9 as in the classic pathway; eventually the lysis of the bacteria can be achieved by the formation of a membrane attack complex (MAC). The mechanism involved in the formation of the MAC will be discussed in Chapter 2.

The activation of the alternative complement pathway has been implicated as a major mechanism in several acute inflammatory reactions which may result in significant tissue damage. Factors that are involved in the activation process are currently considered as potential targets for anti-inflammatory drug design. For example, the development of complement inhibitors such as Nafamostat and other related protease inhibitors may be useful for the treatment of complement mediated disorders and xenograft transplantations.

Collectins are a group of polypeptides in the serum which can bind carbohydrate moieties commonly found only on the surface of microorganisms. For example, one collectin is mannose-binding lectin (MBL) which specifically binds mannose residues on the surface of bacteria. MBL-mannose complexes can interact with collectin receptors on phagocytes and, subsequently, act as opsonins to increase phagocytosis. MBL-mannose complexes can also activate a specific serum protease to initiate the activation of complement components, a process which is similar to the alternative complement pathway. Therefore, collectins can enhance the clearance of microorganisms without the involvement of antibodies. It has been shown that low levels of collectin expression in humans can lead to higher susceptibility to infections, indicating that collectins play important roles in the innate immunity.

Interferons

Interferons (IFNs) are a group of antiviral glycoproteins with molecular weights ranging from 16 to 27 kDa. Depending on the mechanism of their induction and the cells of their production, IFNs can be classified into three types: α-interferon (IFN-α), β-interferon (IFN-β), and γ-interferon (IFN-γ) (Table 1.4). Both IFN-α and IFN-β are induced by viral double-strained RNA; IFN-α is produced by lymphocytes and macrophages while IFN-β is from fibroblasts and epithelial cells. Even though there are at least 20 subtypes of IFN-α and 2 subtypes of IFN-β in humans, genes of both IFN-α and IFN-β are located on chromosome 9 and share an identical receptor. Therefore, IFN-α and IFN-β are sometimes referred to as type 1 IFNs to distinguish from IFN-γ as the type 2 IFN. IFN-γ is produced by T-lymphocytes when stimulated with mitogens such as lectins or foreign antigens to which they have been previously sensitized. Only one type of IFN-γ has been identified in humans; its gene is located on chromosome 12 and its receptor is distinct from that of IFN-α and IFN-β.

IFNs released from virus-infected cells bind receptors on neighboring cells and induce an antiviral state which helps to isolate infective foci. The antiviral activity is most likely a result from the activation or induction of many cellular proteins upon the binding to the IFN receptor. One of the major proteins that becomes activated by the binding of IFN receptor is the enzyme (2′–5′) oligoadenylate synthetase. The product of this enzyme, (2′–5′) oligoadenylate, can activate ribonuclease R which is specific to double strained viral RNA and, thus, can prevent viral propagation inside the target cells. In addition to the activation of virus-specific ribonucleases, IFNs can also induce the synthesis

ANTI-VIRAL ACTIVITY OF INTERFERONS

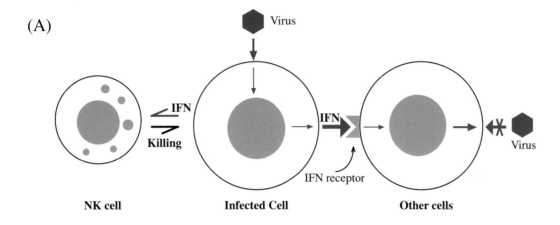

(A)

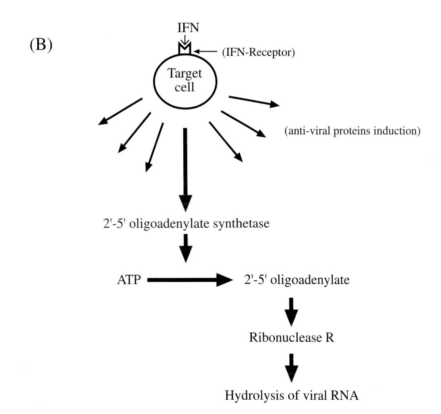

(B)

Figure 1.8. The anti-viral action of interferons. When cells are infected with viruses, interferon synthesis will be induced possibly by the viral RNA, The released interferons send signals to activate NK cells and subsequently, activated NK cells will recognize and kill the virus-infected cells (A). This process can be considered as a self-destructive mechanism in order to prevent the propagation of the viral infection. Interferons can also send signals to other adjacent cells and protect those cells from virus infection. This protection is mediated through the binding of interferons to their receptors (B). Binding of interferon receptors can induce the formation of many anti-viral proteins. One of the major interferon-induced proteins is an enzyme, 2′–5′oligoadenylate synthetase. This enzyme catalyzes the reaction that converts ATP into 2′–5′oligoadenylate,. This unique oligonucleotide can activate a ribonulease which possesses the specificity in the hydrolysis of viral RNA and thus can stop the propagation of virus inside the cell.

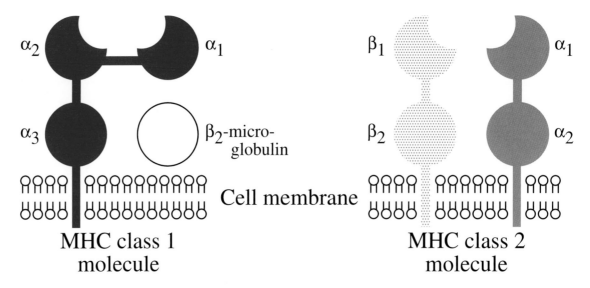

Figure 1.9. The structures of class I and II MHC molecules. The class I MHC molecule consists of a 45,000 daltons polypeptide which has three domains, as indicated α_1, α_2 and α_3. On the surface of the cell, this peptide is non-convalently associated with a molecular weight 12,000 polypeptide β_2- microglobulin which is identical within a species. The diversity of the polypeptide occurs on the area between α_1 and α_2 which is usually referred to as the alloantigenic site. In the class II MHC molecule, it consist of two polypeptides, namely, α (molecular weight 33,00 daltons) and β (molecular weight 28,000 daltons) chains, associated together by non-covalent interactions. The alloantigenic sites are located between α_1 and β_1 domains.

of protein kinase which will inhibit viral protein synthesis inside target cells (Figure 1.8).

Because of their potent antiviral activity, IFNs can be used for the treatment of many diseases caused by viral infection. Recombinant IFNs are now available from several pharmaceutical companies and have been proven to be effective in the prevention of rhinovirus infection and the promotion of recovery from many viral infections including papilloma virus, herpes virus, and hepatitis B virus. However, it should be emphasized here that IFNs have many activities other than the prevention of viral infection. In fact, IFN-γ, also known as immune interferon, is considered to be a factor more important for the regulation of immune system than for its antiviral activity. The other activities which are associated with IFNs are the activation of macrophages, cytotoxic lymphocytes, and anti-proliferative activity against tumor cells. Therefore, recombinant IFN-α has been approved by the FDA for the treatment of several diseases including hairy cell leukemia, AIDS-related Kaposi's sarcoma, and condyloma. In addition, IFN-β has recently been approved for the treatment of multiple sclerosis. IFN-γ is a very potent agent and has been approved or is in trials for the immunotherapy of many diseases. IFN-mediated immunotherapy for cancer and infectious diseases will be discussed in detail in Chapter 7.

The Major Histocompatibility Complexes

The recognition of self and non-self is the foundation for the developement of most immune responses, particularly acquired immunity. This recognition is achieved by the identification of various markers expressed on the surface of cells. There are a group of surface proteins which are the major markers for this recognition; they are referred to as the major histocompatibility complex (MHC) antigens due to their involvement in the compatibility of organ transplantation. For example, the maturation of T-lymphocytes in thymus, as we have briefly mentioned before, involves the screening of immature T-cells for their recognition capability of MHC molecules. Only a small fraction of the thymocytes entering thymus from the bone marrow can fulfill this requirement and will develop into mature T-lymphocytes. In fact, many autoimmune diseases result from the failure of T-cells to distinguish self and non-self MHC molecules. MHC antigens are different classes of proteins in each species; for humans, MHC antigens are expressed from HLA gene clusters located on chromosome 6; they are separated into several subregions as HLA-A, -B, -C and -D. Proteins expressed from HLA-A, -B and -C are class I MHC molecules, and from HLA-D, which contains DP, DQ, and

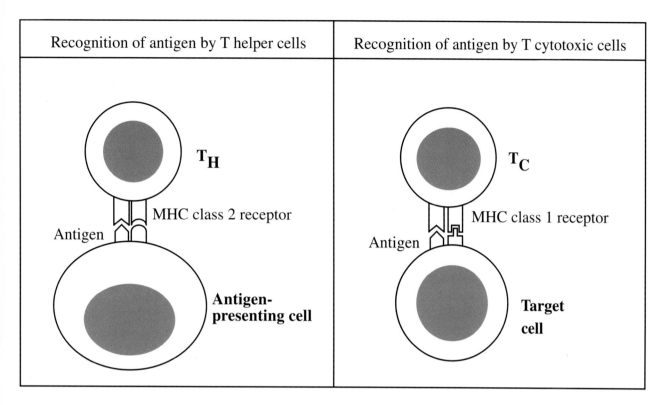

| Recognition of antigen by T helper cells | Recognition of antigen by T cytotoxic cells |

Figure 1.10. The recognition of antigens with MHC molecules. When an antigen is associated with a class I MHC molecule on the cell surface, it is recognized by cytotoxic effector cells, resulting the killing of the antigen-bearing cell, e.g., virus-infected cells. On the other hand, when an antigen is associated with a class II MHC molecule on the surface of antigen-presenting cells, it will be recognized by T helper cells and the antigen will be processed to elicit further response such as the formation of antibodies.

DR subregions, are class II MHC molecules (Figure 1.9). Between class I and II genes, there are regions designated as class III genes; class III genes do not express surface molecules and therefore are not MHC antigens. The high polymorphism observed in both class I and II proteins makes them highly specific to each individual. Proteins expressed from MHC complex with definite specificity are assigned as the locus of the gene followed by a number, e.g., A1, B14 and DR4. A letter "w" which stands for "workshop" is added to names of those protein antigens with currently uncertain specificity, e.g., Aw33, Bw41 and DQw5. There are more than 80 specificities of MHC antigens from human HLA genes that have been identified. Class I

MHC molecules can be found on virtually all nucleated cells in the human body, while class II MHC molecules are only associated with B-lymphocytes and macrophages but can be induced to express on the surface of capillary endothelial cells and epithelial cells. Class I MHC molecules are markers which are recognized by natural killer cells and cytotoxic T-lymphocytes. When class I MHC co-expressed with viral antigens on virus-infected cells will signal as cytotoxic target cells (Figure 1.10). On the other hand, class II MHC molecules are markers indicating a cooperative immune response between immunocompetent cells, e.g., between an antigen-presenting cell and a helper T-cell during the elicitation of antibody formation (Figure 1.10). ■

References

- **Benjamini E, Sunshine G, Leskowitz S.** (1996). *Immunology, A Short Course*, 3rd ed. New York: Wiley-Liss
- **Jenway C Jr, Travers P.** (1994). *Immunobiology – The Immune System in Health and Disease*. New York: Garland Publishing Inc
- **Roitt I, Brostoff J, Male D.** (1996). *Immunology*, 4th ed. Mosby
- **Sell S.** (1996). *Immunology, Immunopathology & Immunity*, 5th ed. Stamford, CT: Appleton & Lange

Journals for Reviews of Current Topics in Immunology

Immunology Today (Elsevier Science Ltd., Oxford, UK)
Current Opinion in Immunology (Current Biology Ltd., London, UK)
Immunological Reviews (Munksgaard, Ltd., Copenhagen, Denmark)
Annual Review of Immunology (Annual Reviews Inc., Palo Alto, CA)

Innate Immunity

- **Bancroft GJ, Kelly JP, Kaye PM, McDonald V, Cross CE.** (1994). Pathway of macrophage activation and innate immunity. *Immunol Lett*, 43, 67–70
- **Baron S, *et al*.** (1991). The interferons: Mechanisms of action and clinical applications. *JAMA*, 266, 1375–1383
- **Kolble K, Reid KB.** (1993). Genetic deficiencies of the complement system and association with disease — early component. *Int Rev Immunol*, 10, 17–36
- **Lehrer RI, Lichtenstein AK, Ganz T.** (1993). Defensins: Antimicrobial and cytotoxic peptides of mammalian cells. *Ann Rev Immunol*, 11, 105–128
- **Rotrosen D, Gallin JI.** (1987). Disorders of phagocyte function. *Ann Rev Immunol*, 5, 127–150
- **Turner MW.** (1996). Mannose-binding lectin: The pluripotent molecule of the innate immune system. *Immunol Today*, 17, 532–540
- **Vose JM, Armitage JO.** (1995). Clinical applications of hematopoietic growth factors. *J Clin Oncol*, 13, 1023–1035

Case Studies with Self-Assessment Questions

Case 1

JR is a 68 year old white male. Approximately two months prior to admission, he began to lose his appetite. Despite several visits to this primary physician, no physiological etiology of cachexia (appetite loss) was determine. Two weeks prior to admission, JR developed spontaneous bruises on his trunk and upper extremities. Furthermore, JR developed persistent gum and nasal bleeding. He was finally admitted into the hospital when he fainted and fell. His admitting diagnosis was pancytopenia due to possible leukemia or lymphoma.

A bone marrow biopsy was obtained revealing a large number of myeloblasts. The working diagnosis was acute myelogous leukemia M3 or acute promyelocytic leukemia. Following confirmation by the attending pathologists, JR was advised to start induction chemotherapy consisting of high dose cytarabine and daunomycin.

He tolerated the chemotherapy with only moderate nausea and vomiting. However, he developed severe neutropenia 4–5 days after the completion of chemotherapy. His clinical course was uneventful till day 10 after chemotherapy, at which time he developed a temperature of 38.6°C. His fevers persisted for 1 hour at which time the medical team started the patient on empiric antibiotics after blood cultures were sent off to the laboratory.

Question 1: Name the various types of granulocytes that circulate in the blood. What are the normal circulating half-lives for the various types of granulocytes?

Question 2: Describe how granulocytes exert their antibacterial activity?

Question 3: Give two clinical options in a patient with neutropenia and febrile neutropenia (fevers that develop during neutropenia)?

Answer 1: Granulocytes are white blood cells that have granules in the cytoplasm. Three types of granulocytes are found in the circulation in human blood: basophils, eosinophils, and neutrophils. Their circulating half-lives are less than 10 hours for neutrophils and unknown for basophils and eosinophils.

Answer 2: Neutrophils are the major bactericidal cells among all granulocytes in the blood.
Neutrophils kill bacteria via phagocytosis process.

Answer 3: Neutrophil development and expansion is primarily dependent on two cytokines, GM-CSF and G-CSF. These two cytokines are now available in recombinant forms as therapeutic agents. Patients who have severe neutropenia (absolute neutrophil counts less than 500 cells/mm³) will have accelerated neutrophil recovery after administration of recombinant GM-CSF or G-CSF. Although both cytokines can be used to accelerate neutrophil recovery, the use of GM-CSF in patients with neutropenic fever is highly discouraged. Administration of GM-CSF in patients with an active infection may potentiate the expression of IL-1 and TNF, which may lead to septic shock.

Case 2

A patient who was diagnosed as having metastatic melanoma and did not respond to conventional chemotherapeutic treatments. Subsequently, recombinant human alpha-interferon (rIFN-α) was selected by his physician as an alternative treatment. After the first I.V. infusion of a recommended dose of rIFN-α at 5×10^6 units/day, the patient developed a fever of 101.3°F and suffered from chills, nausea, and malaise. The physician, however, was optimistic and considered these reactions as an indication of the anti-tumor activity of rIFN-α.

Question 1:   *Do you agree with the physicians prognosis based on this patients reactions to the rIFN-α treatment? Why?*

Question 2:   *The physician plans to continue the treatment by giving the second dose of rIFN-α infusion as originally scheduled. Do you recommend cessation of therapy based on the patients reactions to the first cycle? Why?*

Question 3:   *Do you believe that rIFN-α is a good choice for the treatment of other solid tumors such as lung and breast cancer?*

Answer   1:   Those reactions are general responses of the immune system to interferons and do not necessarily indicate any anti-tumor activity. However, the anti-tumor activity of interferons may be related to the stimulation of the immune system.

Answer   2:   Those reactions to the first cycle treatment are common to interferon therapy and are not life-threatening; therefore, there is no reason to stop the second cycle treatment. However, the patient should be carefully monitored for those symptoms to avoid overreactions.

Answer   3:   rIFN-a is mostly used as a cancer therapeutic agent for virus-caused cancer such as hairy cell leukemia and Kaposi's sarcoma. Its uses for the treatment of commonly occurring solid tumors, such as lung, colon and breast cancer, have not been well established.

2 Antibodies and Complement

As described in Chapter 1, the innate immune response involves various types of cells such as granulocytes and macrophages, as well as many soluble factors such as complements and cytokines. These cellular and humoral factors play the role of first line defense to protect the body from infections. The innate immune response is usually inefficient due to its non-specificity and simplicity. However, upon contact with infectious agents, the immune system can slowly develop another response, i.e., the acquired immune response, which is adaptive to the specific challenge. Therefore, the acquired immune response is more effective in fighting selective infectious agents because of its specificity. Similar to the innate immune response, the acquired immune response can also be divided into cellular immunity and humoral immunity. In this chapter, two of the most important factors, i.e., antibodies and complement, involved in humoral immunity of acquired immune response will be discussed.

Antibodies — The Center of the Humoral Immunity

Antibodies are a group of glycoproteins which are present in serum, as well as in almost all physiological fluids of vertebrates, as immunoglobulins (Igs). The simplest structure of an immunoglobulin molecule consists of two identical short polypeptide chains, the light chains, and two identical long polypeptide chains, the heavy chains, interconnected by several disulfide bonds. All antibodies consist of either κ or λ light chain polypeptides; however, within a single antibody molecule only one type of light chain polypeptide occurs. Furthermore, heavy chain polypeptides within a single antibody molecule are all identical; thus the structure of an antibody molecule is highly symmetrical as shown in Figure 2.1. The two amino terminal regions from one light chain and one heavy chain form a binding site for the antigen. These amino terminal regions of light chains

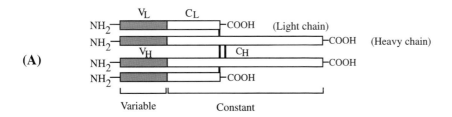

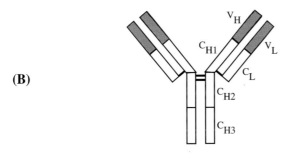

Figure 2.1. The basic structure of an immunoglobulin molecule.
(A) Linear arrangement of the four polypeptide chains with disulfide linkages between a light chain and a heavy chain, and between two heavy chains. Variable regions, where the antigen interaction occurs, are indicated in blue.
(B) Conformational arrangement of the four polypeptide chains as in an immunoglobulin molecule.
VL: Light-chain variable region; CL: Light-chain constant region; VH: Heavy-chain variable region; CH: Heavy-chain constant region.

Property	IgA	IgD	IgE	IgG	IgM
Molecular weight	160,000 or 385,000 (dimer)	184,000	188,000	146,000	970,000 (pentamer)
Heavy chain	α	δ	ε	γ	μ
Light chain	λ,κ	λ,κ	λ,κ	λ,κ	λ,κ
Serum conc. (mg/ml)	4	0.03	0.005	12	1.2
Half-life (days)	6	3	2	23	5
Subclass isotypes	2	1	1	4	1
Carbohydrate (%)	10	13	10	3	10
Complement fixation	No	No	No	Yes	Yes
ADCC	No	No	No	Yes	No
Mucosal secretion	Yes	No	No	No	No
Placenta transfer	No	No	No	Yes	No

Table 2.1. Human immunoglobulin classes.

(V_L) and heavy chains (V_H) are referred to as variable regions. On the other hand, the carboxyl terminal regions of light chains (C_L) and heavy chains (C_H) are referred to as constant regions. The high variation in amino acid sequences in variable regions reflects the large probability of antigen specificity that an antibody molecule can exhibit. The peptide sequence in the center of a heavy chain, as indicated in Figure 2.1(B) between C_H1 and C_H2, is called the hinge region. Hinge regions can provide flexibility for antibodies to bind two separate but identical antigenic structures, or epitopes, with various distances; this flexibility is important for the binding of an antibody to the surface of a target cell.

Antibodies can be divided into several classes. In humans, antibodies consist of five classes: immunoglobulin A (IgA), immunoglobulin D (IgD), immunoglobulin E (IgE), immunoglobulin G (IgG), and immunoglobulin M (IgM) (Table 2.1). The five classes of antibodies differ from each other in the heavy chains of immunoglobulin molecules; for IgA, IgD, IgE, IgG, and IgM the heavy chains are α, δ, ε, γ, and μ, respectively. For example, an IgA molecule consists of α heavy chains with either κ or λ light chains. Each class of antibody has a unique molecular structure and plays a specific role in humoral immunity.

Immunoglobulin A: Immunoglobulin A, IgA, is the major secretory antibody. It is present in dimeric form (Figure 2.2) in almost all physiological fluids such as tears, saliva, gastrointestinal fluids, milk, and other mucus fluids. The two monomeric IgA immunoglobulin molecules are held together by a polypeptide J chain and wrapped by a polypeptide called secretory component (SC). SC is a portion of the IgA-receptor structure on the surface of epithelial cells involving the secretion of this antibody (Figure 2.3). SC polypeptide provides not only an additional linkage besides J chain between the two IgA moieties, but also a protection against proteolysis in the mucosal fluids, especially in the GI lumen. Vertebrates secrete a large amount of IgA, and it is estimated that the human body secretes about 1 g of IgA into its mucosal fluids every day. IgA is also present in the serum at a concentration about 1 to 2 mg/ml; however, unlike the secretory IgA, serum IgA is only monomeric.

IgA is the most important antibody in mucosal immunity. As a secreted antibody in mucosal fluids, IgA can neutralize microorganisms and toxins before those pathogens can enter into or cross epithelia. Furthermore, IgA in the milk can provide neonatal immunity.

Immunoglobulin D: IgD (Figure 2.2) is found predominantly on the surface of B cells. It is present in serum with very low concentrations (<0.1 mg/ml) and short durations (half-life <3 days). The role of IgD in the immune response is not clear, except that it binds antigen molecules on the cell surface to stimulate the activation of the B cells.

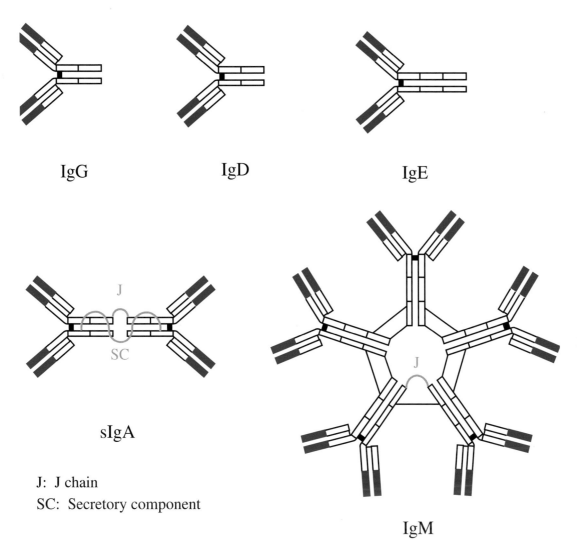

J: J chain
SC: Secretory component

Figure 2.2. Structures of human immunoglobulins. The five classes of immunoglobulin (IgG, IgD, IgE, IgA and IgM) differ from each other on the heavy chains (γ, δ, ε, α, and μ), not only the amino acid sequence, but also the number of domain (4 domains for IgG, IgD and IgA, and 5 domains for IgE and IgM), of the polypeptides. IgM and the secretory IgA (sIgA) are pentamers and dimers, respectively. Some of the IgM may exist as hexamers. There are different J-peptides in IgA and IgM to link the monomers together. In addition, sIgA is protected by a binding peptide, secretory component (SC), which is a fragment of the IgA receptor on the surface of the mucosal cells.

Immunoglobulin E: IgE (Figure 2.2) is found almost exclusively on the surface of mast cells. Upon binding to antigen molecule, IgE can cross-link with each other on the surface of the mast cell and stimulate the release of many allergic mediaters. The role of IgE in allergic reactions will be discussed in Chapter 5.

Immunoglobulin G: IgG (Figure 2.2) is the most predominant immunoglobulin in the serum. Normal serum contains approximately 15 mg/ml of IgG, which is about 75% of total serum immunoglobulin. IgG also possesses the longest half-life of all classes of immunoglobulin in the

blood, i.e., 3 weeks. IgG is capable of crossing the placenta and the immature intestinal epithelium to provide immunity to the fetus and the newborn infant.

IgG is the most important antibody in the serosal immunity. IgG has a high affinity to the antigen and IgG-antigen complexes can be recognized by complement factors and by Fc-receptors on the surface of phagocytes. In both cases, IgG binding leads to the elimination of antigen-bearing cells.

Immunoglobulin M: IgM (Figure 2.2) exists in the blood as a pentamer, and in some cases, as a hexamer. The

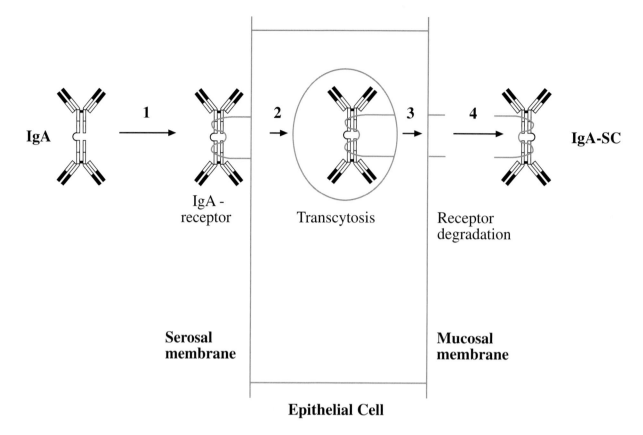

Figure 2.3. The processing of IgA across mucosal epithelium. Dimeric IgA molecules bind to receptors on the serosal side of an epithelial cell. These receptors are called polyimmunoglobulin receptors (pIgR) which are specific to dimeric IgA and, to some extent, to pentameric IgM. Binding to the receptor will transport the IgA from the serosal side to the mucosal side via a vesicular transport mechanism, i.e., transcytosis. On reaching the mucosal side, pIgR will be partially digested and release a fragment of the receptor, the secretory component (SC), with IgA to the lumen. SC can protect the IgA activity from the luminal environment, especially in the lumen of the gastrointestinal tract where proteolytic enzymes are abundant.

polymeric structure is formed by disulfide linkages between the immunoglobulin moieties and a polypeptide J chain. Monomeric IgM is present on the surface of B cells.

IgM is the first antibody produced by the fetus and is also the first antibody to respond when presented with a new antigen challenge. In the primary response against a new antigen, the appearance of IgM in the blood precedes that of IgG. The production of IgM decreases when the production of IgG increases. Therefore, IgM in the serum amounts only about 1.5 mg/mL with a half-life in the blood of less than a week. Usually, the affinity of each antigen binding site in IgM is lower than that in IgG. However, the multivalent attachment of pentameric IgM gives it very high avidity toward the surface of antigen-bearing microbes. Antigen-IgM complex can activate the complement system but, unlike IgG complexes, not macrophage-mediated cytotoxicity.

In addition to these differences between the five classes of immunoglobulin, each class may also exist as different subclass antibodies. In humans, IgG can be separated into four subclasses, i.e., IgG1, IgG2, IgG3, and IgG4. IgA also exists in IgA1 and IgA2 subclasses. Subclasses of immunoglobulin differ from each other in their heavy chain structures. For example, there are four types of heavy chain in human IgG, i.e., γ1, γ2, γ3, and γ4; they are isotypes of the γ-peptide chain.

The difference between classes and subclasses of immunoglobulin is due to the variation in the nature of the heavy chains, i.e., they are essentially different polypeptides. Difference in the nature of polypeptides can also be found in immunoglobulins with identical heavy chain but different light chain, i.e., λ and κ chains. This type of difference in immunoglobulin structures is called isotypic variation. However, immunoglobulins from different individuals may be different due to genetic variations. These changes usually are very minor and involve only one or two amino acids in the constant region of an immunoglobulin molecule. This type of variation is called allotypic variation.

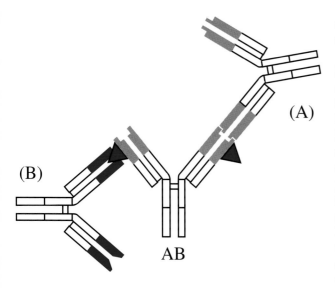

Figure 2.4. Anti-idiotypic antibodies. (A) Private idiotypic antibody: An anti-idiotypic antibody recognizes the antigen-binding site on the variable regions of an antibody, AB. (B) Public idiotypic antibody: An anti-antibody binds to an area on the variable region other than the antigen-binding sites.

These genetic markers usually are not important in the immune response; however, they are important as markers for the study of immunogenetics and for the detection of genetic diseases.

Even among immunoglobulins within an identical isotype and allotype, there are variations between their amino acid sequences at the antigen-binding sites. The segments of polypeptide at the antigen binding site are referred to as variable regions or V-regions. Therefore, unless they are produced from a single clone of B cells, i.e., monoclonal antibodies, there will be differences in the V-regions between any two immunoglobulin molecules. This type of difference in the amino acid sequences of the variable region at the antigen-binding sites is referred to as idiotypic variation (Figure 2.4). An idiotypic variation can be either "private" or "public", depending on whether the difference in the amino acid sequence is located in the antigen-binding site or in other sites of the variable region.

Antibody Fragments

Antibodies can be converted to different fragments of immunoglobulin molecules by treatment with various agents (Figure 2.5). When treated with reducing agents such as dithiothreitol, the disulfide linkages between heavy chains and light chains are cleaved and the antigen binding structure destroyed. However, active antibody molecules can be

reconstructed when a mixture of the reduced light chains and heavy chains is reoxidized.

When treated with proteases without reduction of disulfide linkages, fragments of antibody molecules with an intact antigen-binding capacity can be generated. Papain, a protease isolated from papaya, digests selectively peptide bonds in heavy chains at a position before the disulfide linkage at the hinge region, and therefore, can produce two identical antigen-binding fragments, Fab, and a fragment consisting of only the constant region, Fc. On the other hand, protease pepsin selectively digests a peptide bond after the hinge region disulfide linkage and, therefore, produces two antigen-binding fragments linked by a disulfide bond, F(ab')$_2$. Fab and F(ab')$_2$ are protein fragments with molecular weights only one-third and two-thirds that of an intact immunoglobulin G. They have many advantages when used in diagnostic and therapeutic applications because they are smaller than the intact antibody molecules.

Antigens, Haptens, and Immunogens

A foreign substance which can be recognized by the immune system and can elicit immune responses is called an immunogen. A substance which can elicit the formation of antibodies with a binding affinity toward its specific recognizable structure is called an antigen. Therefore, an antigen is a substance that not only can elicit the formation of, but also can bind to, the induced antibodies. The terms "immunogen" and "antigen" are often used interchangeably. However, strictly speaking, an immunogen may elicit immune responses from cellular immunity without the formation of antibodies. Similarly, an antigen may elicit the antibody formation without any immune response. Since we will discuss the formation of antibodies in this chapter, only the term "antigen" will be used. Not all foreign substances are antigens. To be an effective antigen, the substance must have a large molecular weight. The minimum molecular weight for an antigen is dependent on the nature of the substance; generally, for polypeptides the minimum molecular weight as an antigen is 10 kDa. However, there are small molecules such as N-acetyl-L-tyrosine that are antigens to certain species despite their low molecular weights. In addition to the large molecular weight, an antigen molecule must be capable of being catabolized in antigen-presenting cells. The involvement of antigen degradation in antigen presentation will be discussed later.

The structure of a macromolecule is also important for its antigenic properties. The complexity and steric conformation of an antigen molecule are important factors for the

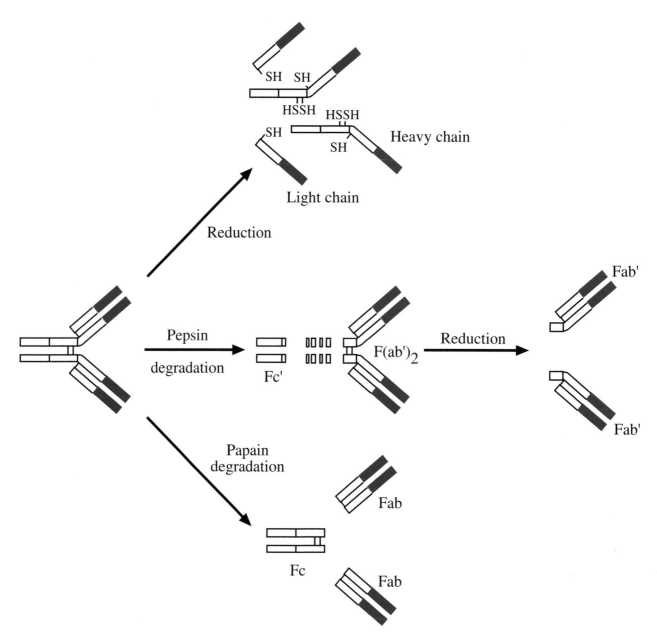

Figure 2.5. Antibody fragments. Antibodies can be reduced to produce two identical heavy chains and two identical light chains. These fragments cannot bind the antigen unless they are oxidized and reconstructed into an intact immunoglobulin. However, antibodies can be digested by proteases, e.g., pepsin and papain, to produce various fragments. Some of the fragments, such as Fab from papain digestion and F(ab')2 and Fab' from pepsin digestion, can maintain the original antigen-binding capacity and are important agents in antibody-mediated therapy or diagnosis.

determination of the effectiveness in eliciting antibody formation, because an antibody recognizes not only the primary sequence of an antigenic macromolecule such as a polypeptide or polysaccharide but also its three-dimensional structure. On the other hand, macromolecules with simple structures such as polyethylene glycol, poly(amino acids), and starch are poor antigens.

When small molecules such as a drug molecule are conjugated to a macromolecular carrier and the conjugates are used for immunization, antibodies can be elicited to recognize and to bind the structure of the macromolecular carrier as well as the conjugated small molecules (Figure 2.6). Those small molecules are not antigens because they cannot induce the formation of antibodies by themselves,

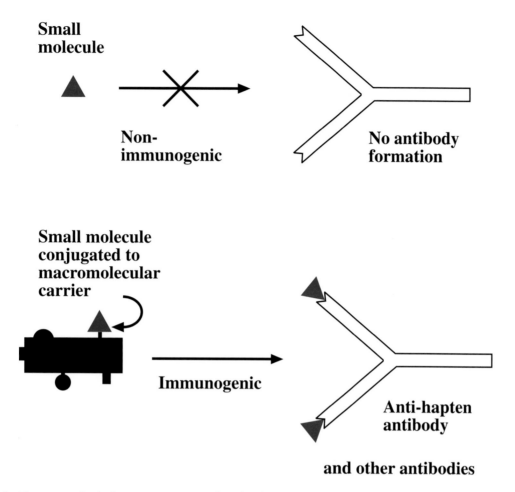

Figure 2.6. Anti-hapten antibody formation. (A) A small molecule is not a covalently linked immunogen and cannot elicit antibody formation. (B) When the small molecule is coupled to an macromolecule, the conjugate is immunogenic and can elicit the formation of various antibodies, including an antibody that recognizes the structure of the small molecule as well as other epitopes on the macromolecular surface.

and are called haptens. Haptens are involved in many drug allergic reactions and are important in the preparation of anti-drug antibodies for the treatment of drug toxicity and for the development of immunoassays in drug analysis.

Antigen Processing and Antibody Formation

Antibodies are produced by B-lymphocytes. In humans, B cells differentiate from stem cells in bone marrow. The differentiation initiates when the immunoglobulin-encoding genes rearrange into a unique sequence which determines the antigen-specificity of the antibody to be produced by the B cell. Upon being stimulated by the specific antigen, the small number of B cells that bear the specific antibody on their plasma membranes will be induced to proliferate into a larger B cell clone. Subsequently, the specific clone of B cells will differentiate into plasma cells and produce only the specific antibody which recognizes the specific antigen (Figure 2.7). Such a clone selection process is also involved in the development of antigen-specific T lymphocytes.

When an antigen molecule enters into the body, it is recognized first by antigen-presenting cells (APC). APC are macrophage-like cells, including Langerhans cells in the skin and dendritic cells in the spleen, which can internalize the antigen molecule via a process called endocytosis. The internalized antigen molecule will be partially degraded into large fragments inside an intracellular compartment, endosomes; those fragments possessing recognizable antigenic structures will be complexed intracellularly with class II MHC proteins and expressed together onto the surface of APC.

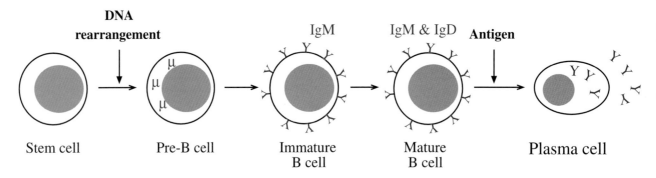

Figure 2.7. B-cell differentiation. Stem cells differentiate into pro-B cells by rearranging immunoglobulin genes, and become pre-B cells when functional immunoglobulin DNA for μ-heavy chains are constructed. This process occurs in the bone marrow and on the surface of stromal cells, involving many cell adhesive molecules (CAMs) and stem-cell factor (SCF) for binding and a stromal cell-secreted cytokine, interleukin 7 (IL-7), for promoting pre-B cell differentiation. The antigen specificity of the B cells is already determined at this stage. Subsequently, after the DNA for light chains also rearranged, the monomeric IgM molecules are assembled and expressed on the surface of immature B cells. Before leaving bone marrow and migrating to peripheral lymphatic tissues such as spleen and lymph nodes, immature B cells must be screened for self-antigen recognition. Immature B cells that express surface IgM recognizing self-antigens inside the bone marrow will be eliminated inside the bone marrow. Once they have migrated to the peripheral tissues, mature B cells express not only IgM but also IgD and IgG on the cell surface. Mature B cells will differentiate into antibody-producing plasma cells and, to a lesser extent, to memory B cells after encountering the specific antigen that is recognized by the surface immunoglobulins.

Antigen fragment-MHC class II complexes on the surface of APC can be recognized by both B- and T-lymphocytes which bear the antigen binding moieties on their surfaces. These surface-bound antigen-recognizing moieties are immunoglobulins for B-lymphocytes and T cell receptors for T-lymphocytes. A B cell and a T cell may bind to an identical antigen fragment but at distinct sites, hence most antigen molecules possess multiple antigenic recognition sites. Furthermore, the binding of both B cell and T cell to the APC surface-bound antigen fragments also involves the simultaneous recognition of class II MHC moiety in the complexes and therefore antigen-presentation by APC is an MHC-dependent process.

The binding of B cells to APC stimulates the secretion of interleukin 1 (IL-1) from APC which induces the differentiation of B cells into the specific antibody-producing plasma cells. The binding of T cells to APC stimulates the secretion of B cell growth factors from T cells which can further promote the proliferation of B cells and the production of antibodies. The antigen-presentation process will be discussed in detail in Chapter 3. Antigen molecules that require the participation of T cells in order to elicit antibody production are called T cell-dependent antigens. There are antigens which do not require the presence of T cells for eliciting antibody formation; these antigens are called T cell-independent antigens (Figure 2.8). T cell dependent antigens are potent antigens and are more effective and sensitive than T cell-independent antigens when they are used for the production of antibodies. In addition to the promotion of B cell proliferation and differentiation, T cells also secrete interleukin 2 (IL-2) which can stimulate the expression of IL-2 receptors on T cell themselves and promote their proliferation to develop cell-mediated immunity.

Antibody Preparation

Antibody preparation is an important sector of the pharmaceutical industry. It consists of low technologies such as antiserum production, to the medium range such as highly purified immunoglobulins, and to high technology such as monoclonal and recombinant antibodies.

Regardless of the technology used for the production of antibodies, the most critical step in most methods is the immunization of animals with a selective antigen. The response of an animal to the immunization depends on many factors other than properties of the antigen molecule as described in Antigens, Haptens, and Immunogens. An antigen molecule must be foreign to the host animals and should be pure enough to avoid the immune response to the contaminating substances. Adjuvants can be used to enhance the immune response. The preparation of immunogens and the use of adjuvants in immunization will be described in detail in Chapter 9 Vaccines. The response of an animal to immunization also depends on factors in the host animal such as the age, sex, genetic strain, and physical condition. In addition, the location and the method of

(A) T cell-dependent antigens

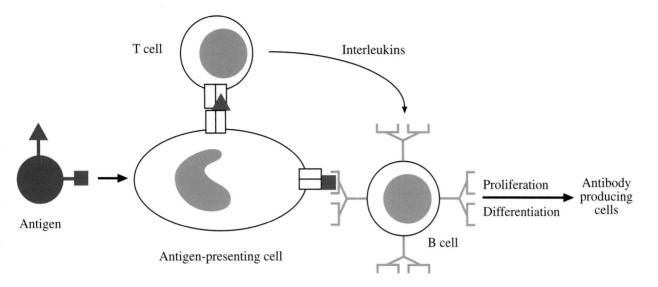

(B) T cell-independent antigens

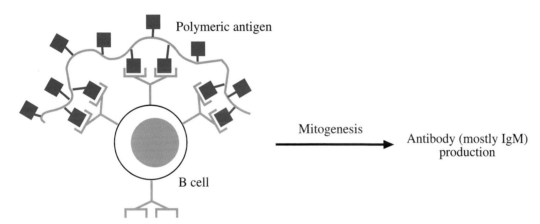

Figure 2.8. The processing of T cell-dependent (A) and T cell-independent (B) antigens. T cell-dependent antigens usually consist of more than one antigenic determinants. After processing by antigen-presenting cells (APC), the surface-expressed, MHC-complexed antigen determinants will be recognized by the antigen-specific B and T cells. T cells will release interleukins, e.g., IL-4 and IL-6, which will induce the proliferation and differentiation of B cells into antibody-producing plasma cells. T cell-independent antigens, such as a polymeric antigen with repeating determinants, can bind directly to the immunoglobulins on the surface of a B cell. This type of cross-binding on the cell membrane, often in the presence of other mitogens, will induce the proliferation and differentiation of the B cell. T cell independent antigens usually elicit the production of only IgM antibodies with low titers.

injection can determine the type and extent of the immune response.

The amount of a specific antibody in the serum is presented as the titer of the antibody. The titer usually refers to as the extent of dilution of the serum in which the antibody still can be detected by conventional immunological techniques. The titer and the class of antibodies in the serum are both dependent on the schedule of the immunization. In the primary immunization, i.e., when the host is exposed to the antigen for the first time, the titer is

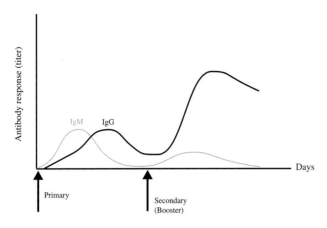

Figure 2.9. Primary and secondary antibody responses. When a host is exposed to an antigen for the first time, i.e., the primary antigenic challenge, a lag time for several days is usually observed for the immunity to begin the production of antigen-specific antibodies. This primary response usually produces IgM first followed by a low titer of IgG, and only lasts for a short period of time. When the host is exposed to the same antigen again, i.e., the secondary antigenic challenge, antibody production occurs in a very short time and is predominantly IgG. The secondary response of antibody production not only is with higher titers but also lasts much longer than the primary response.

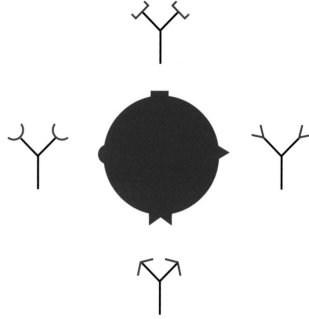

Figure 2.10. Polyclonal antibodies are produced by many different clones of B cells which can recognize different epitopes on the surface of an antigen molecule. As illustrated in this figure, different antibodies recognize various shapes of epitope on a spherical antigen. Therefore, polyclonal antibodies such as antisera isolated from immunized animals are essentially mixtures of many types of antibodies with regard to the classes of immunoglobulin and the specificity and affinity toward antigens.

usually very low. Furthermore, the class of antibodies from the primary response is predominately IgM. In the secondary immunization, that is when the animal is challenged or boosted with the antigen for the second time, the response is relatively fast; the titer of the antibody increases markedly and the class of the antibody shifts from IgM to IgG (Figure 2.9). Several booster injections may be required in order to obtain serum with desirable titer and specificity. However, an overboosted animal may produce antiserum with a decrease in both the titer and the specificity.

When serum of an immunized animal is used as a source of antibodies, it consists of many antigen-binding immunoglobulins with different specificity and produced from many different clones of B cells (Figure 2.10). Therefore, this type of antibody is called polyclonal antibody.

Another method for the production of antibodies is by using hybridoma technology (Figure 2.11). In this method, a small animal such as a mouse is first immunized with a selected antigen. When the serum obtained from the animal after boost injections indicates a high titer of antibody against the selected antigen, the animal will be sacrificed and cells will be isolated from the spleen. The splenic cells contain a large number of B-lymphocytes; at least some of the B-lymphocytes can produce the antigen-specific antibodies. The isolated splenic cells, because they are normal cells, have a very short life in cultures. How-

ever, these cells can be fused with transformed cells such as myeloma cells in the presence of fusogens such as polyethylene glycol to produce half-normal-half-transformed cells, which are called hybridomas. If a hybridoma is formed by the fusion between an antibody-producing B-lymphocyte and a myeloma cell, this hybridoma will possess both the antibody production capability of a B cell and the unlimited proliferation ability of a cancer cell. After careful selection of the fusion products, a single clone of hybridoma can be picked and propagated. This clone of hybridoma will continuously produce a single type of antibody as regards the specificity and class of immunoglobulin. This type of antibody is called monoclonal antibody because it is produced by a single clone of B-lymphocyte.

A comparison of the properties of polyclonal and monoclonal antibodies is shown in Table 2.2. The choice of either a monoclonal or a polyclonal antibody depends largely on the purpose of the use. If the purity and specificity of the antibody is important such as the use of antibody as a drug, monoclonal antibodies are usually preferred. On the other hand, if the affinity and costs of the antibody are important, such as the use of an antibody as an analytical

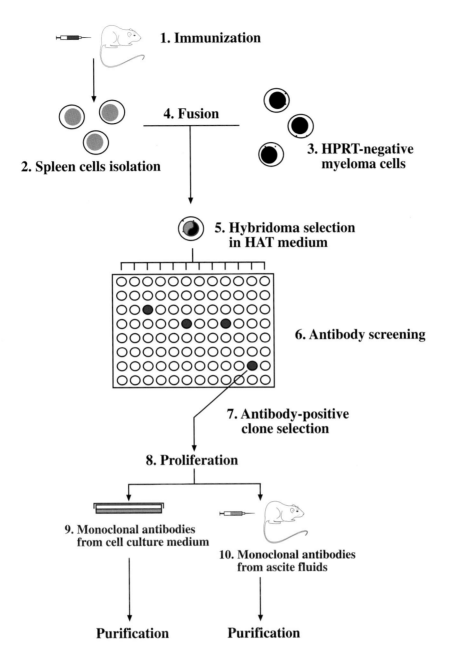

1. Immunization

4. Fusion

3. HPRT-negative myeloma cells

2. Spleen cells isolation

5. Hybridoma selection in HAT medium

6. Antibody screening

7. Antibody-positive clone selection

8. Proliferation

9. Monoclonal antibodies from cell culture medium

10. Monoclonal antibodies from ascite fluids

Purification

Purification

Figure 2.11. Monoclonal antibody production. 1. Mouse is immunized with the specific antigen. 2. After anti-antigen antibody can be detected in the serum, mouse will be sacrificed and spleen cells will be isolated. Spleen cells consist of a large number of B cells. 3. A myeloma cell line is selected which is deficient in the enzyme hypoxanthine-guanine phosphoribose transferase (HPRT). This cell line cannot survive in a medium containing aminopterin, a thymidine synthetase inhibitor, because the cell cannot use purines in the salvaged pathway for DNA synthesis. 4. The spleen cells and the HPRT-negative myeloma cells are fused in the presence of fusogens such as polyethylene glycol. 5. After fusion, cells will be maintained in a medium containing hypoxanthine, aminopterin and thymidine (HAT). Only cells that are fused between one spleen cell (with enzyme HPRT) and one myeloma cell (immortal), i.e., a hybridoma cell, can survive in the HAT medium. 6. Hybridomas will be diluted and seeded in small well plates (e.g., 96-well microtiter plates) with one cell per each well. After many days in culture, each well will have enough cells for the screening of the production of antibodies. 7. Wells that produce desirable antibodies will be identified. 8. Cells in those wells will be transferred and proliferated into a large number of hybridoma cells. 9. The culture medium will contain a high concentration of the monoclonal antibody against the specific antigen. If necessary, the antibody can be purified to homogenity by using various immunoglobulin isolation techniques such as affinity chromatography. 10. For large scale production, the hybridoma cells can be injected intraperitoneally into mice, and the ascite fluids can be collected and, if necessary, purified to obtain the monoclonal antibody preparation.

Properties	Polyclonal	Monoclonal
Preparation	Simple	Complicated
Purification	Impure	Pure
Specificity	Variable and multiple	Consistent and single
Isotype	Mixture	Single
Stability	Stable	Uncertain
Affinity	High	Uncertain
Quantity	Limited	Unlimited

Table 2.2. Comparison of polyclonal and monoclonal antibodies.

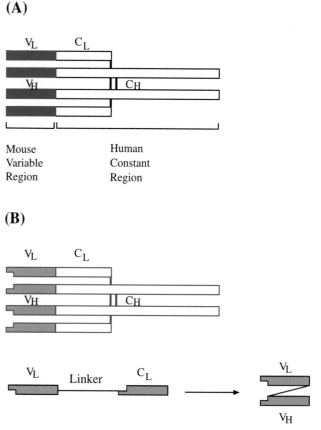

(A)

Mouse
Variable
Region

Human
Constant
Region

(B)

Figure 2.12. Examples of antibodies produced by genetic engineering technology. (A) Chimeric antibodies with mouse variable regions and human constant regions are produced by recombinants of mouse and human immunoglobulin cDNA's. By substituting the Fc region in a mouse immunoglobulin, e.g., a mouse monoclonal antibody, by a human counterpart, the antigenicity of the mouse immunoglobulin will be greatly reduced in the human immune system. (B) Fv fragments cannot be obtained by degradation of immunoglobulins because there is no disulfide linkage to hold the two polypeptides together. However, recombinant DNA technology can produce single chain Fv polypeptide (sFv) which consist of VL and VH peptide sequences connected by a linker peptide which provide a linkage of the two polypeptides without interference of the antigen-recognition activity.

agent in immunoassay, polyclonal antibodies are usually the choice.

In addition to the production from serum and hybridomas, antibodies can also be made by using the recombinant technology. Two of the most important features for the development of recombinant antibodies are (1) the preparation of chimeric or humanized antibodies that consists of human constant regions to minimize the hypersensitization to animal immunoglobulins in patients (Figure 2.12), and (2) the preparation of single chain Fv fragments (sFv) that possess antigen-binding capability with a minimum molecular weight of approximately 25 kDa, i.e. half of that of Fab fragments (Figure 2.12).

Genetic Basis of Antibody Diversity

It has been estimated that in humans there are at least 10^7 types of antigenic structures that can be recognized by the immune system. This large diversity of antibody specificity has been a puzzle for immunologists for many years, and many theories have developed for its explanation. It is only during the last ten years that, due to the advent of modern molecular biology, immunologists have finally been able to understand the genetic basis that control the diversity of antibody formation in B cells. However, many mechanisms involved in the antibody formation such as the class switch and the fine tuning of specificity are still not fully understood at the present time.

The most important event in antibody biosynthesis is the rearrangement of genes to form DNA sequences which upon expression, transcription and translation, will produce specific antibodies. This process involves DNA rearrangement and RNA splicing leading to a specific light chain or heavy chain. Therefore, for each light or heavy chain, its encoded DNA is presented as many segments within a cluster of genes on a specific chromosome which is chromosome 2 for κ, chromosome 22 for λ, and chromosome 14 for heavy chain.

For κ-light chain, there are three regions of genes which encode the polypeptide sequences, i.e., V, J and C regions. V and C regions correspond to the variable and constant regions in the polypeptide chain, and J (joining) region

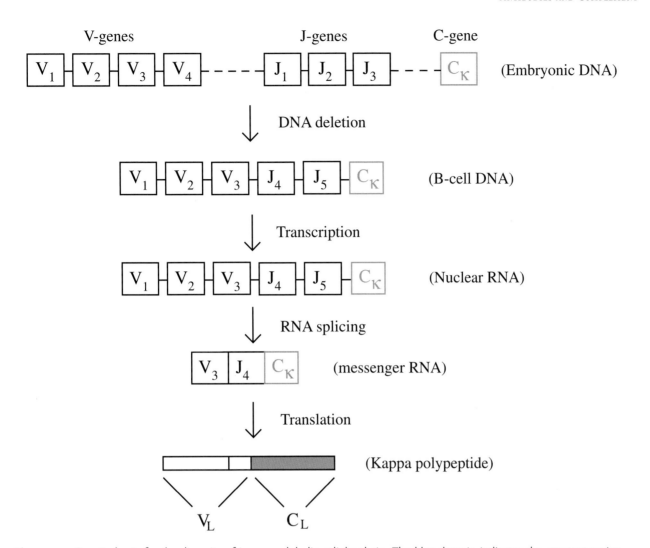

Figure 2.13. Genetic basis for the diversity of immunoglobulin κ-light chain. The blue domain indicates the constant region and the white domains indicate the variable region. The specificity of the immunoglobulin is determined as early as in the DNA deletion process; for example, the linking of V_3 and J_4 segments will determine the antibody specificity as shown in this diagram.

encode a small peptide segment which joins the V and C peptides to form the complete light chain. In human B cells, there are 200 V genes, five J genes, and one C gene for a κ-chain. Therefore, a total of 1,000 different combinations for κ-chain structures can be synthesized (Figure 2.13). A similar process is also responsible for the large number of combination for the formation of λ-chains.

For heavy chains, there are four regions of genes encode the polypeptide. In addition to the V, J, and C regions, there is a D (diversity) region of small segments of genes which can be inserted between V and J regions to further increase the diversity of the heavy chain amino acid sequence. In human B cells, there are approximately 150 V genes, 12 D genes and four J genes. In addition, there are nine C genes that encode the nine isotypic variations of the heavy chain, i.e., μ, δ, γ_3, γ_1, α_1, γ_2, γ_4, ε, and α_2.

The combination of the variable regions (V+D+J) can produce approximately 7,200 different structures of the heavy chain. Because the heavy chain and light chain are encoded in different genes and in different chromosomes, their pairing to form an immunoglobulin molecule is random. Therefore, when a light chain and a heavy chain combine together to form an antigenic binding site (Fab), there are approximately 7.2 million combinations, and thus 7.2 million types of antigen specificity can be produced. In addition, the C region genes can also rearrange to form different classes or subclasses. This rearrangement, known as class switch, occurs after the completion of the rearrangement of VDJ gene of the heavy chain, and is determined by other factors, e.g. interleukin-4 (IL-4) and transformation growth factor-beta (TGF-β) in the process of the immune response.

In addition to the gene rearrangement and light chain-heavy chain combination, the diversity of antibody can also be generated from point mutation of gene. This mutation usually occurs in the hypervariable regions by altering one amino acid residue that leads to a marked increase of the affinity toward the antigen.

Complement

Antibodies are factors in the humoral immunity for the recognition of pathogens via antibody–antigen interaction.

In very few cases, antibody-binding on the surface of target cells alone can cause the killing of the antigen-bearing cells. However, in most cases, subsequent events are required in order to generate cytotoxicity and to destroy the target pathogens. One of the mechanisms involved in antibody-mediated cytotoxicity is by complement activation which causes the lysis of the target cells.

Complement factors are a group of serum proteins which are designated by symbols as C1 to C9. Once the activation of complement factors is initiated, the cascade will proceed to form a complex, i.e., membrane attack complex (MAC), on the surface of the target cell which will cause lysis of the

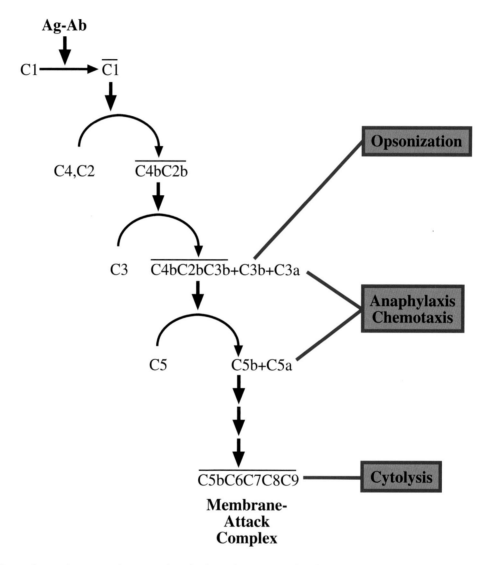

Figure 2.14. Classical complement pathways and its biological activities. The classical complement pathway is initiated by the binding of C1 factor to the antigen-antibody complexes of IgG or IgM. The enzyme cascade (C1 to C5), followed by a sequential aggregation (C6 to C9), will form a membrane-attack complex (MAC) which is a cylindrical transmembrane pore and is capable of lysing the antigen-bearing target cell. Binding membrane-fixed C3b fragments can induce the phagocytosis of the target cells by C3b-receptor bearing phagocytes, a process referred to as opsonization. In addition, the release of C3a and C5a fragments can attract phagocytes to the inflammatory site via chemotactic effects, and cause anaphylaxis via binding to endothelium and mast cells. A bar above the components indicates an active complex.

cell membrane. As described in Chapter 1, the innate immune response can initiate the complement cascade, a process which is called the alternative complement pathway. However, in acquired immunity, the complement cascade is initiated by the interaction of complement factors with antibody–antigen complexes, and this process is called the classical complement pathway. A comparison of these two complement pathways has been described in Figure 1.7 in Chapter 1.

There are nine factors involved in the classical complement pathway (Figure 2.14). Functionally, these nine factors can be divided into two categories of proteins: proteins with proenzymatic activities such as C1, C2, C3, and C4, and proteins with aggregating activities such as C5, C6, C7, C8, and C9. During the complement cascade, factors C1 to C5 require enzymatic transformation into the active forms while factors C6 to C9 do not need activation.

In the classical complement pathway, the Fc domain of an antigen-bound antibody can be recognized by complement protein C1. C1 protein consists of six C1q subunits with six binding sites at one end held together by the six long fibrous peptides at the other end; an arrangement resembles six tulips held together by tying the six stems. In addition, there are two C1r and two C1s molecules associated with the "stem" structure. The six C1q binding sites can interact with the Fc domains (C_H2 and C_H3) of antibody–antigen complexes formed by all subclasses of IgG molecules, except IgG4. The six binding units in C1q can form a crosslinkage between two IgG molecules. IgM molecules are the only isotype of immunoglobulins other than IgG's that are also recognized by C1q. Because IgM molecules consist of five immunoglobulin units, C1q can bind more than one Fc (C_H4) domain in each IgM molecule.

Upon C1q binding to the Fc portion of an antigen-bound IgG or IgM molecule, C1r proenzyme is activated. Activated C1r subsequently converts C1s to an active enzymatic form and initiates the cascade in the classical complement pathway. C4 is the first complement component in the blood which is activated by C1s. C4 is split into two polypeptides, the shorter one is C4a and the longer one is C4b. C4b, as an activated enzyme, can convert complement C2 component into a larger polypeptide with enzymatic activity, C2b, and a shorter polypeptide, C2a. C2b and C4b form a complex with C1s on the antigen-bearing surface, known as C3 convertase, which can convert C3 into C3a and C3b. As can be seen in Figure 1.6 in Chapter One, the formation of C3b is an important step in both the alternative and the classical complement pathways. C3b binds to the membrane with antibody–antigen complex and can enhance the phagocytosis of the target cell by phagocytes via the C3b receptors present on the surface of the phagocytes. The process of enhancing phagocytosis by the attachment

Opsonin	Binding Receptor	Phagocytosis
No	No	Poor
Antibody	Fc Receptor	Fair
Complement	C3b Receptor	Fair
Antibody and complement	Fc + C3b Receptors	Good

Table 2.3. Effects of opsonization on phagocytosis.

of marker molecules on the surface of the target cells is called opsonization. The marker molecules recognized by phagocytes are opsonins. Besides C3b, antibody–antigen complexes when bound to the surface of target cells can also behave like opsonins by enhancing phagocytosis via Fc receptors on the surface of phagocytes (Table 2.3).

The membrane-bound complex of C4b,C2b,C3b is called the C5 convertase which produces a membrane-bound C5b fragment by cleaving off a small C5a fragment from the C5 component. During the activation process from C1 to C5, three small polypeptide fragments are generated, i.e., C3a, C4a, and C5a. Although these three small peptides *are not directly involved* in the complex formation on the surface of target cells that eventually produce the cell death, they are important factors for the induction of inflammatory responses. C4a, C3a, and C5a are anaphylatoxins because they bind to mast cells and basophils and stimulate the release of granules from these cells. The degranulation of mast cells or basophils releases several important inflammatory mediators including histamine. These mediators cause the anaphylatic response: the contraction of smooth muscles and leakage of the endothelium. These anaphylatoxic peptides are inactivated by an anaphylatoxin inhibitor, carboxypeptidase B, in the serum which removes the carboxyl terminal arginine residue. In addition to the anaphylaxis, C5a also acts as a factor of chemotaxis and an activator of neutrophils (see Chapter 1). However, the chemotactic activity of C5a is not reduced by the action of carboxypeptidase B.

Unlike factors C1 to C5, complement components following C5b in either the classical or the alternative pathway do not require modification or activation. Thus, intact C6, C7, and C8 molecules aggregate sequentially around C5b to form a membrane-associated complex which, in turn, polymerizes C9 molecules to form a transmembrane channel. This transmembranous channel, known as the membrane attack complex, consists of an average of 15 molecules of C9 and acts as a pore to cause the leakage of electrolytes and other cytoplasmic components from the antigen-bearing cells. Eventually, the target cells are killed by this cytolytic action. ∎

References

- **Bogue M, Roth DB.** (1996). Mechanism of V(D) J recombination. *Curr Opin Immunol*, **8**, 175–180
- **Chen J, Alt FW.** (1993). Gene rearrangement and B-cell development. *Curr Opin Immunol*, **5**, 194–200
- **Davies DR, Sheriff S, Padlan EA.** (1988). Antibody–antigen complexes. *J Biol Chem*, **236**, 10541–10544
- **Esser C, Radbruch A.** (1990). Immunoglobulin class switching: Molecular and cellular analysis. *Ann Rev Immunol*, **8**, 717–735
- **Honjo T, Alt FW, eds.** (1995). *Immunoglobulin Genes*, 2nd ed. San Diego: Academic Press
- **Miletic VD, Frack MM.** (1995). Complement-immunoglobulin interactions. *Curr Opin Immunol*, **7**, 41–47
- **Morgan BP.** (1995). Physiology and pathophysiology of complement: progress and trend. *Crit Rev Clin Lab Sci*, **32**, 265–298
- **Owens RJ, Young RJ.** (1994). The genetic engineering of monoclonal antibodies. *J Immunol Meth*, **168**, 149–165
- **Raag R, Whitlow M.** (1995). Single-chain Fvs. *FASEB J*, **9**, 73–80

Case Study with Self-Assessment Questions

Scientists in your biotech company have identified a specific marker, BX, from biopsy tissues of human breast cancer patients. The Company is interested in developing an anti-BX antibody for the potential applications in breast cancer diagnosis and treatment. BX has been characterized by the Chemistry Group in the Company as a glycopeptide with a molecular weight of 2,500 daltons. When BX-human serum albumin conjugate was used as an immunogen, anti-BX antiserum was obtained from immunized rabbits. Preliminary results from screening of patients' blood samples using rabbit anti-BX antiserum indicated a positive correlation between the level of BX and breast cancer occurrence. The Company decided to immunize mice with BX-conjugate for the production of monoclonal anti-BX antibodies for further development of breast cancer diagnostic kits and, potentially, breast cancer immunotherapeutic drugs.

Question 1:   *Why was BX conjugate, instead of BX itself, used as an immunogen to produce antibodies? Why was human albumin, instead of rabbit albumin, used for the preparation of the conjugate?*

Question 2:   *What are the possible immunoglobulin isotypes present in the rabbit antiserum as anti-BX antibodies?*

Question 3:   *Why did the Company decide to produce monoclonal anti-BX antibodies instead of using the current anti-BX antiserum for new product development.*

Answer 1:   The effectiveness of an antigen to elicit antibody formation is dependent on many factors. BX, with a molecular weight of 2.5 kDa, is too small to be an antigen. In order to produce an antibody that will recognize the structure of BX, this small glycopeptide must be linked to a large molecular carrier as a hapten immunogen. The macromolecular carrier should be foreign to the host species. When rabbits are used as hosts for immunization, rabbit proteins such as rabbit albumin should not be used as immunogens.

Answer 2:   The anti-BX antiserum produced from the immunization of rabbit is a polyclonal antibody which consists of all possible classes of rabbit immunoglobulins including IgG, IgM and IgA.

Answer 3:   Monoclonal antibody technique can continuously produce a large quantity of pure and well-characterized immunoglobulins. These criteria are important especially if the antibodies are to be used in therapeutic applications. However, monoclonal antibodies usually do not possess the high affinity and high cytotoxicity of polyclonal antibodies, and sometimes they are less stable than antiserum. Furthermore, mouse monoclonal antibodies when used as therapeutic agents may elicit the formation of anti-mouse immunoglobulin antibodies (HAMA) in humans. Genetic engineering technology can make chimeric antibodies, humanize antibodies, and single chain Fv fragments (sFv) that are potentially superior to mouse monoclonal antibodies as therapeutic agents.

3 Cellular Responses in Immunity

As described in Chapter 1, all circulating cells found in the blood are derived from the same pool of parental cell or pluripotent stem cells (PSC). The pluripotent stem cell is primarily found in the bone marrow of long bones and the pelvis. Although these PSC make up only 0.1% of all the cells found in the marrow, these are the cells that give rise to all circulating blood cells (Figure 3.1).

Unlike any other cells, PSCs have the capacity to undergo asymmetric mitosis or "Self Renewal." During this process, the stem cell divides into two daughter cells. One

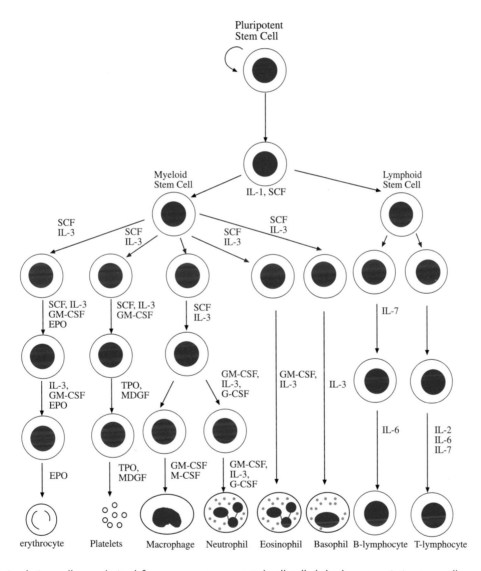

Figure 3.1. All circulating cells are derived from a common parental cell called the hematopoietic stem cell or pluripotent stem cell. In this diagram, the evolution of the various circulating cells is influenced by the various cytokines that regulate their maturation and differentiation process.

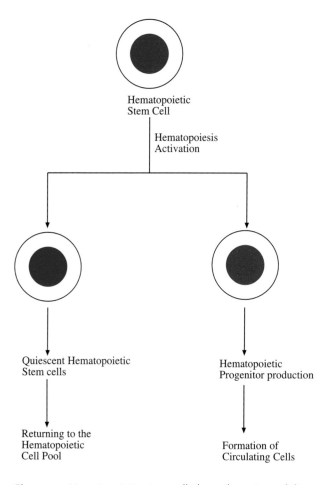

Figure 3.2. Hematopoietic stem cells have the unique ability to "Self Renew", whereby the formation of two daughter cells results in the formation of circulating cells. However, one of these daughter cells will retain its quiescent state and rejoin the pool of stem cells, thus maintaining the same number of parental cells.

daughter cell will mature and differentiate to form circulating cells, whereas the other daughter cell will retain its quiescent state, and rejoin the pool of stem cells, thus maintaining the same number of parental cells (Figure 3.2).

The differentiation and maturation process into mature circulating cells is under the control and regulation of hematopoietic cytokines or growth factors. These cytokines may also determine the type of circulating cell formed. Activated stem cells can evolve into either myeloid or lymphoid cells. The process as to how the progenitor cell knows what type of cell to form is still unclear. Progenitor cells are pluripotent and can differentiate into a lymphoidal progenitor cell. The maturation of lymphoid progenitor cells is influenced by lymphokines which determine whether the progenitor will form either T- or B-lymphocytes. On the other hand progenitor cells that are programmed to form myeloid cells will form either erythrocytes, platelets, monocytes/macrophages, or granulocytes (e.g. neutrophils, basophils, and eosinophils).

Cells in the Circulation

Each cell plays an important role in maintaining homeostasis. The various cells found in the circulation are listed in Table 3.1. There are various types of lymphocytes and they are divided into either bursa- (B) or thymus- (T) lymphocytes. B-lymphocytes or plasma cells produce and secrete antibodies, which are used to neutralize foreign invaders and serve as a chemoattractant for cellular elements of the immune defense.

T-lymphocytes can be further divided into either regulatory or effector cells. Regulatory T-lymphocytes can be subclassified as either helper T-cells (T_H: activate the immune system) or suppressor T-cells (T_s: downregulators of

Types of Cells	Biological Activity
Erythrocytes	Oxygen and carbon dioxide transport
Platelets	Clot formation
Neutrophils	Phagocyte to defend against bacterial and fungal infections
Eosinophils	Granulocyte responsive to allergens and parasitic infections
Basophils	Granulocyte responsive to allergens
Macrophages	Phagocyte responsible for antigen presentation and defense against bacterial and fungal infection
Cytotoxic T-lymphocyte	Defense response against viral infection, tumors, and allograft
B-lymphocytes	Antibody producing cells
Natural killer cells	Response against tumor and viral infection

Table 3.1. Peripheral blood cells.

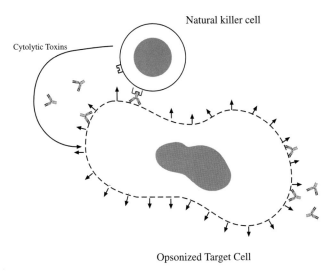

Natural killer cell

Cytolytic Toxins

Opsonized Target Cell

Figure 3.3. Antibody dependent cellular cytotoxicity (ADCC) is where antibody binding will initiate cellular cytotoxicity. Effector cells like natural killer cells (NK) have Fcγ receptors, which allow attachment to antibodies that bind onto pathogenic organisms.

immune response). Helper T-lymphocytes are also referred to as T4 or CD4$^+$ lymphocytes because of the presence of these surface markers. In contrast, suppressor T-lymphocytes that downregulate the immune system bear T8 or CD8$^+$ surface markers.

The effector cells such as cytotoxic T-lymphocytes (CTLs) and natural killer cells (NK) are responsible for eradication of virally-infected or tumor cells. Although the origin of NK cells is still uncertain, the role of NK cells is to eliminate antibody coated pathogen by antibody dependent cell-mediated cytotoxicity (ADCC). NK cells have IgG receptors or Fcγ receptors, which allow attachment to antibodies that have coated the pathogenic organisms (Figure 3.3). NK cells are not phagocytic in nature, rather they carry out their cytotoxic function through formation of perforin complexes that allow the leakage of intracellular contents. Presently, the exact mechanism by which NK cells exert its cytotoxic activity is still unclear.

Most CTLs express CD8$^+$ surface markers, where the T-cell receptor (TCR) recognizes MHC class I molecules instead of MHC class II which are present on APCs. CTLs eliminate cells that express foreign antigens on their surfaces, such as virus-infected host cells and tumor cells. In order for a CTL to acquire cytotoxic activity, it must receive two signals. The first signal is the induction of high affinity IL-2 receptors, which is followed by IL-2 binding onto these receptors, thus initiating cellular cytotoxic activity.

CTLs exert their cytotoxic activity by binding onto target cells that bear MHC class I molecules. After cellular binding, the CTLs will release specific proteins that assemble

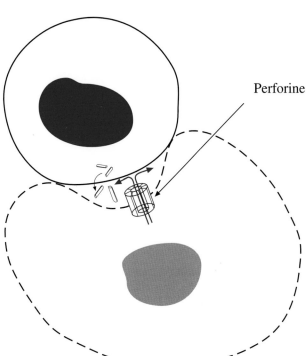

Cytotoxic T-Lymphocytes

Perforine

Targeted Cells

Figure 3.4. The mechanism of cytotoxic T-lymphocyte (CTL) is shown in this figure. CTLs will bind onto the pathogen via T-cell receptors that are specific for antigen. The presence of MHC I will indicate to the CTLs that the organism is indeed foreign, and thus will release a series of cellular toxins that will eliminate the intruder.

on the cellular membrane. This protein complex will form a pore-like channel that will permit intracellular contents leakage, resulting in cellular death (Figure 3.4). CTLs can also activate a sequence of biological signals that can induce intracellular signals that can lead to a process called "apoptosis" which is also known as programmed cell death. Unlike cellular cytotoxicity, apoptosis is where the chromosomes are fragmented by the activation of cellular endonucleases.

Myeloid cells have a wider variety of biological activities. Erythrocytes or red blood cells (RBCs), due to the presence of hemoglobulin which give rise to its red pigmentation, transport oxygen from the lungs to the tissues, and remove the oxidative byproduct, carbon dioxide. Platelets are derived from megakaryocytes, and are important in the repair of vascular damage, through initiation of the coagulation cascade during vascular integrity breakdown.

The remaining myeloid cells are referred to as either granulocytes or monocytes due to their morphology. Granulocytes are so called because of pigmented granules found in the cytoplasm of these cells. Granulocytes are multi-lobed nucleated cells, which is in contrast to macrophages that have an unsegmented nucleus and are often referred to as monocytes (immature macrophages). Granulocytes and monocytes are responsible for cellular response to the presence of antigen.

Eosinophils have granules loaded with histamine which is released during allergic reactions. Release of histamine will result in vasodilation and pulmonary constriction. In addition, eosinophils provide host defense against parasitic infections. Similar to eosinophils, basophils provide inflammatory response to allergic reactions but the exact role of these cells is still unclear.

The other important granulocyte is the neutrophil, which plays a seminal role in the defense against bacterial infections. When the population of neutrophils is reduced below 500 cells/μL, these individuals are susceptible to life-threatening infections. Most notable of these infections is gram-negative bacteremia, which is responsible for the majority of deaths associated wth severe neutropenia.

Macrophages are antigen presenting cells (APCs), which break down the antigen to an identifiable form for immune recognition. Macrophages are sometimes referred to as "scavenger cells" because they remove particles and organisms from the circulation, and are essential in the eradication of bacterial and fungal infections.

Host Defense Mechanism

The body is constantly bombarded with infectious agents, however in the immunocompetent host, only a small percentage of these pathogens actually enter into the circulation and cause clinical symptoms. This is due to the various defense mechanisms, which when functioning normally, will enable the host to maintain a sterile environment.

Barrier defense apparatus such as the skin and mucosal membrane represent the largest mechanism preventing the entrance of pathogens into the circulation. Once the pathogens have evaded the barrier defense, the body will mount an attack consisting of both humoral and cellular immunity. Although the immune system is divided into cellular and humoral compartments, it works in concert to orchestrate an attack that will preserve sterility. The humoral immunity includes neutralizing antibodies and the complement cascade. Additionally, humoral mediators include stimulatory cytokines, such as interleukin-1 (IL-1) and tumor necrosis factor (TNF) will activate immune cellular response. These immunological defenses are summarized in Table 3.2.

• Antigen binding via immunoglobulin or complement factors
• Phagocytosis of antigen by surveillance cells
• Antigens are processed and presented to T-lymphocytes along with MHC class II
• Surveillance cells such as macrophages activate T-lymphocyte via secretion and production of IL-1 and TNF
• Activated T-lymphocyte begins production and secretion of IL-2

Table 3.2. Immune response to antigen presentation.

Antigen Presentation

Once an antigen or a foreign organism has penetrated the barrier defense, non-specific circulating antibodies and complement factors will coat the foreign substance. This coating process is also known as "Opsonization," which serves two purposes; 1) neutralizes the antigen and 2) activates chemotaxis of cellular components. Antibodies and/or complement factors bounded onto pathogens will produce a structural conformational change that results in cellular chemotaxis to the affected site.

The first cell that arrives at the affected site is usually an APC, such as a macrophage or primed B-lymphocyte. These cells have Fcγ and C3b receptors on the cell surface, thus allowing the binding onto opsonized antigen. The opsonized particle is phagocytosed by the macrophage and processed by proteolytic enzymes into smaller fragments, because helper T lymphocytes (CD4$^+$ cells) can only recognize antigens when they are presented on the membrane of the APC. In order for the T-lymphocytes to recognize the antigen, MHC class II protein must also accompany the processed antigen (Figure 3.5).

Once the antigen is processed, this will activate macrophage expression of cytokines. The processed antigen along with the MHC II molecule is then presented to a naive T-lymphocyte, which will activate the cell to upregulate expression of interleukin-2 (IL-2). Along with antigen presentation, IL-1 and TNF are produced by macrophages, which are required to co-stimulate naive T-lymphocytes.

The activation of naive T-lymphocytes will increase expression of IL-1, which will serve as both a paracrinic and autocrinic factor. Paracrinic factors are stimulatory cytokines that are produced by neighboring cells. Whereas autocrinic factors are factors that are produced by the cell, which can also be utilized by the cell itself to further enhance its proliferation and/or stimulation.

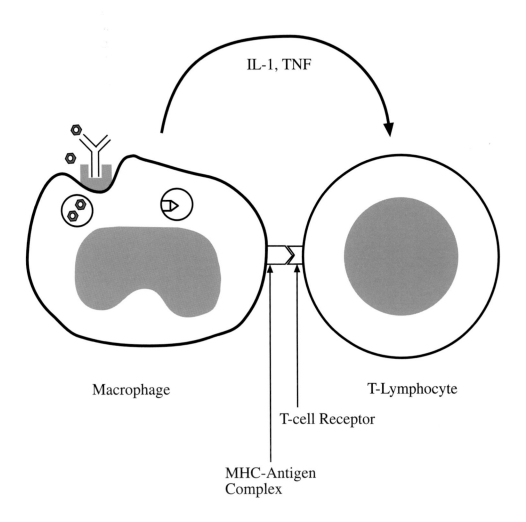

IL-1, TNF

Macrophage

T-Lymphocyte

T-cell Receptor

MHC-Antigen
Complex

Figure 3.5. Antigens that have evaded the barrier defense are neutralized by humoral factors such as antibodies and complement factors. Antigen binding will activate cellular migration to the affected site. Cells such as macrophages with Fcγ and C3b receptors will phagocytose the antigen and degrade it using lysosomal enzymes. The processed antigen is then presented to a naive T-lymphocyte, and is activated by a secondary signal such as cytokine activation.

There are various monocyte-derived cytokines. Most notable are the primary inflammatory mediators like IL-1 and tumor necrosis factor-alpha (TNF-α). CD4⁺ cell activation will in turn initiate immune activation, resulting in autosynthesis of IL-1 and expanding the population of commited progenitor stem cells. Additionally, activated-CD4⁺ cells also produce interleukin-2 (IL-2) which will expand the population of helper-T-lymphocytes, cytotoxic T-lymphocytes, suppress T-lymphocytes, natural killer cells, and B-lymphocytes.

IL-1 is a primary inflammatory mediator that can stimulate the active recruitment of cells to the affected site. There are two ways this can be accomplished. One mechanism is through the demarginalization of immune cells that adhere onto the walls of the endothelium of the microvasculature. The other method is to stimulate maturation

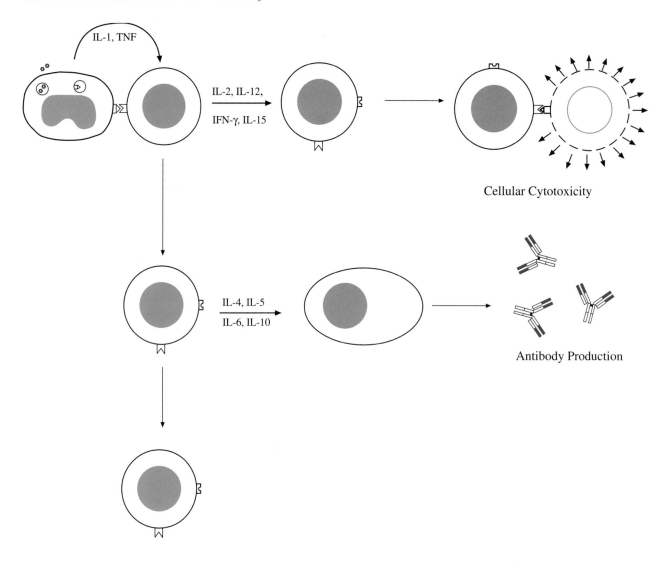

Figure 3.6. There are two populations of Helper T-lymphocytes (T$_H$), which are designated as T$_{H1}$ and T$_{H2}$. T$_{H1}$ regulate cellular immunity responses such as mobilization and expansion of CTLs, whereas T$_{H2}$ regulate humoral immune responses such as increased levels of antibodies and complements factors. The regulation of cellular immunity is controlled by T$_{H1}$, through the expression of IL-2, IL-12, and IFN-γ. These cytokines will modulate CTLs and NK cells, where IL-2 and IL-12 will increase their cytotoxic effects, respectively. IFN-γ is a cytokine that is synergistic to both IL-2 and IL-12, and is able to increase expression of MHC I on target cells.

and differentiation of stem cells to differentiate and expand to form circulating cells. In addition, IL-1 is also able to induce expression of CSFs and lymphokines, which regulate the differentiation, proliferation, and maturation of myeloid and lymphoid cells, respectively.

The activation of T-cell will also enhance the expression of IL-2, which was originally named T-cell growth factor (TCGF). IL-2 is a pleiotropic factor that can activate CTLs, T$_H$ lymphocytes, T$_S$-lymphocytes, B-lymphocytes, and NK cells (Table 3.4). The expression of IL-2 receptor or IL-2R

is one indicator that the cells are activated. In order for IL-2 to exert its activity, it must first bind onto a receptor which activates a series of intracellular signals that will result in cellular activation.

There are two populations of T$_H$ cells that are designated as T$_{H1}$ and T$_{H2}$. T$_{H1}$ regulate cellular immunity, whereas T$_{H2}$ regulate humoral immunity. The regulation of cellular immunity is controlled by T$_{H1}$, through the expression of IL-2, IL-12, and IFN-γ (Figure 3.6). These cytokines will modulate CTLs and NK cells. In addition, IL-2 and IL-12 will increase their cytotoxic effects. IFN-γ is a cytokine that can act synergistically with both IL-2 and IL-12, and is able to increase expression of MHC I on target cells.

In contrast, T_{H2} regulate humoral immunity through expression of IL-4, IL-5, IL-6, and IL-10 (Figure 3.6). IL-4 is able to induce the production of T_{H2} cells, such as eosinophils, and mast cells. In addition, IL-4 will promote IgE expression, suggesting that it plays an important role in allergic reactions. Either IL-4 or IL-10 are able to suppress the induction and function of T_{H1} cells, which may be the mechanism of downregulating cellular immunity.

Role of Cytokines in Immune Response

Following antigen processing, there is release of primary inflammatory response mediators such as IL-1 and TNF. These cytokines not only stimulate the release of IL-2, but also increase recruitment of immunological cells and stimulate the release of local chemotactic agents. Other biological effects of IL-1 and TNF are summarized in Table 3.3. Additionally, TNF and IL-1 are both able to stimulate accessory cells such as fibroblasts, endothelial, and activated T cells to produce other cytokines such as colony stimulating factors (CSFs).

IL-1 is able to mobilize progenitor cells into the peripheral blood compartment, which can mature into circulating lymphoidal or myeloidal cells. Monocyte-derived IL-1 has an autocrinic effect which includes induction of

• Endogenous pyrogen reaction
  – Hypotension
  – Appetite loss
  – Malaise
  – Arthralgias
  – Myalgias
  – Chills and fevers

• Induces the release of kinins and prostaglandins
• Increase permeability of vascular via degradation of basement membrane
• Increase expression of inflammatory cytokines
• Recruit cellular elements to the affected site

• Induce the production of adrenocorticotropic hormone (ACTH)
  – Induce expression of β-endorphines
  – Induce expression of corticosteroids

Table 3.3. Biological activity of tumor necrosis factor and IL-1.

• Increase natural killer (NK) and cytotoxic T-lymphocyte (CTL) activity

• Increase the production and secretion of the following
  – Macrophage: IFN-γ
  – T-lymphocytes: GM-CSF, IL-3, IL-1 and TNF

• Enhance B-cell production of antibodies directed against antigens
• Increase T-suppressor cells which will ultimately turn off immune response
• Enhance expansion of both myeloid and lymphoid cells

Table 3.4. Biological activity of interleukin-2.

IFN-γ receptors, adhesion protein expression, and MHC expression.

The expansion, proliferation, and differentiation of myeloid cells are under the strict control of colony stimulating factors (CSFs). CSFs are classified by their capacity to sustain the proliferation and differentiation of various myeloid progenies in colony forming unit (CFU) assays (Figure 3.7). These factors are designated as granulocyte-macrophage-CSF (GM-CSF), multi-lineage-CSF (Multi-CSF), granulocyte-CSF (G-CSF), macrophage-CSF (M-CSF), erythropoietin (EPO) and thrombopoietin (TPO).

Primarily produced and secreted by either activated T-lymphocytes or macrophages, however endothelial cells and fibroblasts have also been described as producing CSFs. These glycoproteins have variable molecular weights which are dependent on the degree of glycosylation. With the exception of macrophage-CSF, CSFs are single chain molecules with intrachain disulfide bond(s); the disulfide bond(s) must be intact for full biological activity.

Other means to classify CSFs have been to divide them according to their potential biological activity (Table 3.5). They are classified as either pluripotent or unipotent CSFs. Pluripotent or Class I CSFs such as multi-CSF or interleukin-3 (IL-3) and GM-CSF, possess stimulatory activity in a wide variety of lineages and are required throughout the maturation process. In contrast, unipotent or Class II CSFs, such as G-CSF, M-CSF, TPO and EPO, are able to influence only one or two lineages. An important caveat is that all CSFs have been shown *in vitro* to possess the capacity to stimulate the proliferation and expansion of other lineages; this is usually concentration dependent.

The active GM-CSF molecule consists of a single chain 127 amino acid polypeptide, that was derived from a 147 amino acid precursor protein. The secondary structure of the molecule is maintained by two internal disulfide

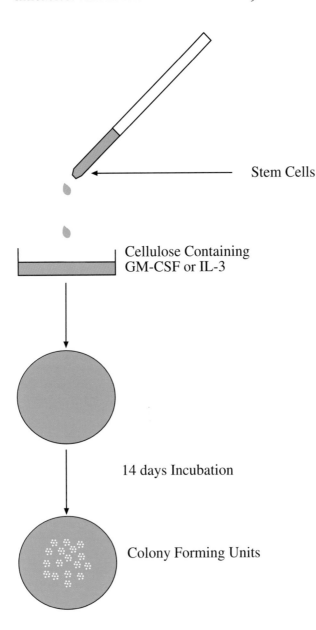

Stem Cells

Cellulose Containing
GM-CSF or IL-3

14 days Incubation

Colony Forming Units

Figure 3.7. Colony forming assays are performed by adding purified bone marrow cells into a semi-solid medium containing either agarose or methylcellulose. Growth factors such as hematopoietic growth factors IL-3 or GM-CSF are required to stimulate clonogeneic colony formation. Within 7–14 days, distinctive hematopoietic colonies are formed.

linkages. Depending on the degree of glycosylation, the molecular weight of GM-CSF ranges from 14-35 kDa.

GM-CSF has unique regulatory activity, enabling it to influence a wide variety of progenies. The biological activity of GM-CSF overlaps with M-CSF and G-CSF to ensure the formation of functional monocytes and granulocytes, respectively. Although *in vitro* studies suggested that GM-CSF

has the capacity to maintain megakaryocytic, eosinophilic, and erythroid lineages, these results have not been confirmed in clinical studies.

Unlike GM-CSF, the regulatory activity of IL-3 is limited to the earlier stages of differentiation and maturation. *In vitro* studies have shown that upon co-receptor binding with another CSF, IL-3 can downregulate other CSF receptors. This downregulation of other CSF receptors may be the mechanism by which progenitor cells are selected into a specific differentiation pathway.

IL-3 is primarily produced and secreted by activated T-lymphocytes and macrophages. It has a molecular weight of 14-28 kDa. Secondary structure is influenced by the presence of a single disulfide bond. Carbohydrate complexes are anchored onto the two arginine residues found in its 133 amino acid polypeptide backbone.

In contrast to the pluripotent CSFs, Class II CSFs regulate differentiation on more mature progenitors. M-CSF is a heavily N-glycosylated dimer that exists as either a soluble or membrane-bound glycoprotein. Its biological activity is lost following reduction of the homodimer, yielding two identical monomeric polypeptides with a MW of 15 kDa each. Three forms of M-CSF have been reported: they have 256, 554, and 438 amino acids and are designated as alpha, beta, and gamma, respectively. Both GM-CSF and IL-3 have overlapping activities with M-CSF in the maturation of monocyte progenies.

The average circulation life span of neutrophils is estimated to be less than about 10 hours. Therefore to maintain basal levels of neutrophils, at least 6 billion new neutrophils must be formed daily. G-CSF is a Class II CSF working in conjunction with both pluripotent CSFs to regulate neutrophil levels. Similar to other CSFs, G-CSF is a single chain polypeptide consisting of 174 amino acids with one internal disulfide bridge. The primary amino acid sequence of G-CSF does not include any arginine linked carbohydrate sites; thus only O-glycosylation appears in this molecule. G-CSF is able to support the maturation of granulocytic progenitors in colony forming unit (CFU) assays. It is also, to a lesser extent, able to support monocytic, megakaryocytic, and erythroid progenies at higher concentrations.

Similar to other blood components, erythrocyte production is under the strict regulation of CSFs. There are various cytokines that regulate the differentiation of early erythroid progenitor cells such as IL-3 and interleukin-11. However terminal maturation into red blood cells is under the control of erythropoietin (EPO). Human erythropoietin is a 30 kDa glycoprotein with 165 amino acids and four carbohydrate side chains. EPO originates from peritubular cells, possibly fibroblasts that are found in the renal cortex. Trace amounts of EPO can be produced from parenchymal cells in the liver. Endogenous EPO production is regulated

Myeloid Growth Factors	CFU-GM	CFU-GEMM	CFU-E	BFU-E	CFU-Meg
M-CSF	+	−	−	−	−
G-CSF	+	−	−	−	−
EPO	−	−	+	+	−
TPO	−	−	−	−	+
GM-CSF	+	+	−	−	−
IL-3	+	+	−	−	+

Table 3.5. Activity of colony stimulating factors.

by oxygen tension, where low levels of oxygen will induce kidney cells to synthesis EPO. Unlike other CSFs, full glycosylation of EPO is required for biological activity. Furthermore, EPO have both N- and O-glycosylation, unlike other CSFs which have one or the other but not both.

Megakaryocytopoiesis is regulated by a number of cytokines with overlapping biological activity. However, the elusive cytokine that regulates terminal differentiation of platelets could not be isolated for 35 years. Although a factor regulating platelet formation was suspected, not until recently was this cytokine isolated and its gene cloned. It was initially called c-Mpl-ligand. cMpL is product of the c-mpl protooncogene, and is the cytokine receptor belonging to the hematopoietin receptor family. This receptor is expressed on megakaryocytes and platelets. Initially this cytokine had various names which included Mpl-ligand (Mpl-L), thrombopoietin (TPO), and megakaryocyte growth derived factor (MGDF).

The TPO gene was located on the long arm of human chromosome 3. Genetic analysis suggests that TPO had a polypeptide backbone consisting of 332 amino acids with striking homology to erythropoietin throughout the N-terminal half. Recombinant TPO has profound effects on megakaryocyte growth and development. These effects appear to include the expansion of megakaryocyte progenitors and induction of megakaryocyte maturation to functional platelet.

It is evident that the maturation, proliferation and survival of circulating blood cells are controlled by the combination of various CSFs. IL-3 and GM-CSF seem to overlap and synergize with each other in their influence on less mature progenies, whereas unipotent CSFs like M-CSF, G-CSF, EPO, and TPO appear to control differentiation in latter stages. It is thus apparent that circulating myeloid cells require both Class I and Class II CSFs to form normal functioning circulating cells. ■

References

- **DiPiro JT.** (1997). Cytokine networks with infection: mycobacterial infections, leishmaniasis, human immunodeficiency virus infection, and sepsis. *Pharmacotherapy*, **17**(2), 205–23

- **Goodman JW.** (1994). The Immune Response. In *Basic and Clinical Immunology Eight Edition*, edited by DP Stites, AI Terr, TG Parslow. Norwalk, Connecticut: Appleton & Lange, pp. 40–49

- **Imboden JB.** (1994). T-lymphocytes and Natural Killer Cells. In *Basic and Clinical Immunology Eight Edition*, edited by DP Stites, AI Terr, TG Parslow. Norwalk, Connecticut: Appleton & Lange, pp. 94–104

- **Louie S, Jung B.** (1993). Clinical effects of biologic response modifiers. *Am J Hosp Pharm*, **50**, S10–18

- **McKinstry WJ, Li CL, Rasko JE, Nicola NA, Johnson GR, Metcalf D.** (1997) Cytokine receptor expression on hematopoietic stem and progenitor cells. *Blood*, **89**(1), 65–71

- **Metcalf D.** (1989). The molecular control of cell division, differentiation commitment and maturation in haemopoietic cells. *Nature*, **339**, 27–30

- **Metcalf D.** (1988). Haemopoietic growth factors. *Therapeutics*, **148**, 516–519

- **Metcalf D.** (1997). The molecular control of granulocytes and macrophages. *Ciba Found Symp*, **204**, 40–50

- **Moldawer LL, Copeland EM 3rd.** (1997). Proinflammatory cytokines, nutritional support, and the cachexia syndrome: interactions and therapeutic options. *Cancer*, **79**, 1828–39

- **Murtaugh MP, Baarsch MJ, Zhou Y, Scamurra RW, Lin G.** (1996). Inflammatory cytokines in animal health and disease. *Vet Immunol Immunopath*, **54**, 45–55

Self-Assessment Question

Question 1: *JQ comes into the emergency room with chills, fever, and rigors. He tells you that he has been experiencing these symptoms the last 3 days. However, he states that he was not around anyone with colds or flu-like symptoms for at least 7 days. Can you explain the lag period when JQ was initially exposed in comparison with onset of symptoms?*

Answer 1: Although JQ was probably infected 7 days ago when he came into contact with infected individuals, symptoms normally do not develop immediately. This may be attributed to the time required for the pathogenic organism to by-pass the barrier defense (e.g. skin and muscosal) and enter the circulation. Once the foreign intrusion has occurred, immunological response must ensue.

   Fevers, chills, and rigors occur because macrophages and activated lymphocytes produce interleukin-1 and tumor necrosis factors, which can induce pyrogenic effects. In order for the clinical signs to occur, enough immune stimulus is required. Two factors can occur here, 1) the pathogen burden on the body, and 2) immune response to the intrusion. The lag time may occur because time is required for the pathogens to replicate and induce an immune response.

4 Antibody as Drug and Drug Carrier

Since conceived by Paul Ehrlich at the turn of the century, for the potential applications in chemotherapy, antibodies have been dubbed as *magic bullets* due to their high specificity and affinity towards pathogenic antigens. However, the therapeutic applications of antibodies became realistic only after the introduction of monoclonal antibodies and the advances of biotechnology in recent years. Several antibodies have already been produced and marketed by pharmaceutical companies as therapeutic drugs for the treatment of human diseases. It can be anticipated that more antibodies, particularly genetically engineered antibodies or antibody derivatives, will be introduced as new drugs in the next few years.

Generally, antibodies can be considered as therapeutic agents in two ways: as drugs and as drug carriers. From the description of humoral and cellular immunity in previous chapters, we should recognize that there are many obstacles when using antibodies for the treatment of various diseases. There are general limitations of using antibodies as therapeutic agents (Table 4.1). However, there are additional limitations that are associated only with the use of antibodies either as drugs or as drug carriers (Table 4.2).

Limitations	Problems
Impermeability of endothelium to antibody molecules	Inaccessible to target tissues
Poor tissue penetration of antibodies	Inaccessible to entire tissue
Antigen heterogeneity and modulation	Ineffective to antigen-negative or antigen-modulated cells
Lack of specific antigen on target cells	Side effects to normal cells
Lack of human monoclonal antibodies	Hypersensitivity towards animal immunoglobulins

Table 4.1. General limitations in antibody therapy.

	As Drugs	As Drug Carriers
Antibody isotype	Isotype dependent	Isotype independent
Antibody modification	Intact antibody	Antibody conjugation
Host immunity	Dependent on host immunity	Independent on host immunity
Target	Antigen-bearing cells	Can be designed to kill bystanding non-antigen cells.
Internalization	Internalization of surface bound antibodies is not required	Internalization is required for most drug–antibody conjugates

Table 4.2. Comparison of antibodies as drugs and as drug carriers.

Antibodies as Drugs

There are two major uses of antibodies for the treatment of human diseases:

Antibodies as Drugs to Neutralize and Eliminate Pathogenic or Toxic Molecules

As stated in Chapter 2, the natural function of antibodies is primarily to bind antigen molecules and to form antigen–antibody complexes. These complexes are cleared rapidly from the blood via either the reticuloendothelial system or, if small Fab fragments are used, the kidneys. Such a process can eliminate selectively the pathogens or toxic substances from the blood or tissues. When using intact antibodies as neutralizing agents in the treatment of human diseases, type III hypersensitivity (serum sickness) is one of the major adverse reactions. This type of hypersensitivity will be discussed in Chapter 5.

Traditionally, antibodies have been used in the form of antiserum to save lives from severe infections or poisoning. For example, rabbit antisera against snake venoms are effective antidotes for poisonous snake bites and anti-diphtheria toxin antisera are used for the treatment of diphtheria infection. It must be emphasized that antigen–antibody complex formation may not result in a total elimination of pathological events. In fact, recent attempts by several biotechnological companies to produce monoclonal antibodies against endotoxins from gram-negative bacteria for the treatment of sepsis and bacteremia in humans have not been very successful.

One of the applications of antibodies as neutralizing agents is for the treatment of drug toxicity. In this case, antibodies are raised against drug molecules as haptens. The preparation of anti-hapten antibody has been discussed in Chapter 2. Both polyclonal and monoclonal antibodies are suitable for this use. Fab fragments are more practical than the intact antibody because they are smaller in size and therefore, their toxic drug complexes can be excreted from the kidneys. Consequently, the half-life of Fab fragments in the blood circulation is much shorter than that of the intact antibody. In humans, the plasma half-life of Fab fragments from a foreign source such as an animal antibody or a mouse monoclonal antibody is approximately 9 hours, which is significantly shorter than that of the intact IgG, i.e. 2 to 3 days. Besides the pharmacokinetic advantages, the dose of antibody required for neutralizing a certain amount of a toxic substance is another important factor to be considered. Due to the relatively large molecular weight of antibody (150 kDa for IgG and 50 kDa for Fab) as compared to toxic substances (less than 1 kDa for most drugs), a large quantity of antibody or Fab fragments must be used in order to bind stoichiometrically the toxic agent in the blood or tissues. Theoretically, Fab fragments can be used at a lower dose than that of the intact antibody. Another advantage of using Fab as a drug is that this fragment is less immunogenic than the intact antibody, and, therefore, is less likely to develop hypersensitive reactions if the treatment has to be repeated in the future.

The most successful example of using antibody to neutralize toxic substances is the treatment of digoxin poisoning which could be either accidental or intentional overdose. Several pharmaceutical companies have marketed digoxin-specific Fab fragment from animal immunoglobulin or monoclonal antibody as an antidote of digitalis poisoning. The Fab fragment is given by i.v. infusion over a period of 30 minutes at a dose of approximately 500 mg per patient, depending on the blood level of digoxin. Free digoxin in the serum of the patient completely disappears during the infusion. However, protein-bound digoxin concentration actually increases rapidly which is due to the removal of tissue-associated digoxin by anti-digoxin Fab. The half-life of the protein-bound digoxin in the serum is approximately 20 hours.

Antibodies as Drugs to Eliminate Target Cells

Antibodies themselves are not inherently cytotoxic and their binding to target cell membrane antigens usually does not directly cause cell death. However, there are four possible mechanisms that antibody-binding can lead to cell death or growth inhibition (Figure 4.1).

REGULATORY GROWTH CONTROL

Antibodies may interfere with the accessibility of essential growth factors to the target cells. This effect can be achieved when an antibody binds to either a growth factor or its cell surface receptor. This approach is particularly attractive in cancer therapy because it is generally believed that many tumor cells produce growth factors as autocrines that stimulate their own proliferation. Antibodies against these autocrine growth factors or receptors for tumor cell proliferation conceivably could inhibit selectively the growth of the tumor (Figure 4.1Aa). Recent studies on the immunotherapeutic applications of anti-HER-2/neu antibodies in breast cancer treatment is an example of this type of antibody-mediated cell growth control. HER-2/neu, an oncogene product that is overexpressed on the surface of most breast cancer cells, is a growth factor receptor, and the binding of antibody to HER-2/neu can regulate the growth of the HER-2/neu-positive breast cancer.

Alternatively, antibody binding on surface markers may promote the differentiation of tumor cells to normal cells and therefore is potentially useful in differentiation therapy. This approach has been proposed for the treatment of B-cell lymphomas. An anti-idiotypic antibody, which recognizes

46

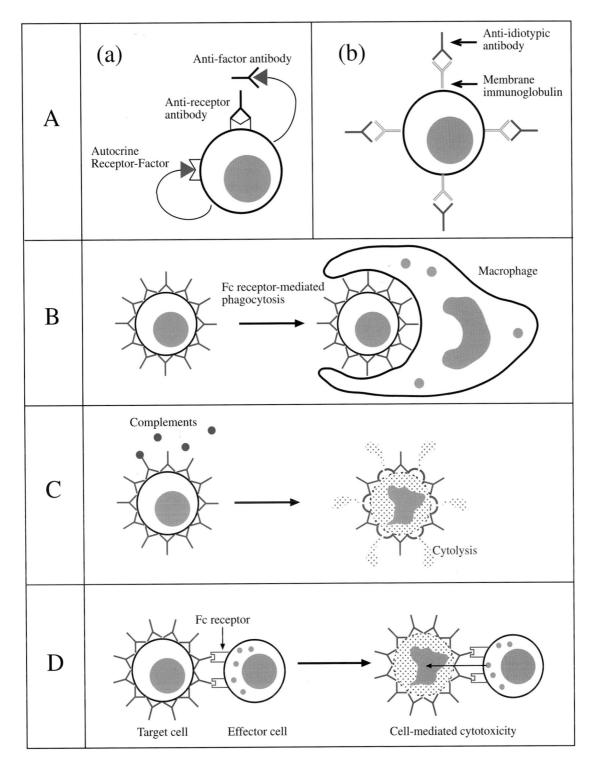

Figure 4.1. Mechanisms of antibody-mediated cytotoxicity. (A). Regulatory growth control: Antibodies against growth factors or receptors, such as autocrine growth factors in tumor cells, can inhibit cell proliferation. Alternatively, anti-idiotypic antibodies against B-cell surface immunoglobulins may induce the differentiation of the B-cell and subsequently, induce their differentiation into plasma cells. (B). Reticuloendothelial clearance: Antibody-binding on the surface of the target cells can enhance the phagocytosis by macrophages, a process of opsonization which is mediated via Fc receptors. (C). Complement-mediated cytotoxicity: Complement fixation can cause the lysis of antibody-bound target cells. (D). Antibody-dependent cell-mediated cytotoxicity (ADCC): The binding of antibody-bound target cells to effector cells such as K cells via Fc-receptor can cause the death of the target cells due to releasing cytotoxic factors from the effector cells.

and binds the variable region of immunoglobulin molecules on a B-lymphoma cell, may mimic the action of an antigen molecule to promote the differentiation of the lymphoma cell into an antibody-producing cell. Such a differentiation process may terminate the proliferation of B-lymphoma cells (Figure 4.1Ab).

RETICULOENDOTHELIAL CLEARANCE

Antibody-coated target cells can be engulfed by phagocytes, mostly macrophages in the reticuloendothelial system (RES), via phagocytosis. Antibodies facilitate the phagocytic process by opsonizing the target cells for either Fc or C3b receptors on the surface of phagocytes, a process that has been described in Chapter 2 (Figure 4.1B).

COMPLEMENT-MEDIATED CYTOTOXICITY (CMC)

Antibodies, either IgG or IgM, when bound to antigen molecules on the surface of target cells can initiate the classic complement pathway as described in Chapter 2. This complement activation can cause the cytotoxicity to the target cells by the formation of membrane attack complex (Figure 4.1C).

ANTIBODY-DEPENDENT CELL-MEDIATED CYTOTOXICITY (ADCC)

Antibody-bound target cells can be recognized by killer cells or macrophages via Fc-receptors and subsequently killed by cell-mediated cytotoxicity. The mechanisms involved in this killing process most likely involve cell–cell contact and the releasing of cytotoxic substances from the effector cell to the target cell (Figure 4.1D). ADCC is considered to be the major function of macrophages or K cells in killing of tumor cells because the size of these target cells is too large to be phagocytosed by RES cells.

Commercial Antibodies Used as Drugs for Prevention or Treatment of Human Diseases

HUMAN IMMUNOGLOBULINS

Human immunoglobulins are obtained from pooled human plasma either of donors from the general population or of hyperimmunized donors. Human immunoglobulins obtained from the general population can be used for the treatment of patients with immunodeficiency syndrome and for the prevention of infection in patients with chronic lymphocytic leukemia. Immunoglobulins obtained from healthy donors, e.g., Gammagard® (Baxter Biotech), Sandoglobulin® (Sandoz), and N-Gamimune® (Miles Biologicals), are intravenous immunoglobulin solutions, or IGIV. They provide immediate antibody levels in the patient's blood with a half-life of approximately three weeks.

Human immunoglobulin solutions containing a high titer of antibody to hepatitis B surface antigen can be prepared and purified from the plasma of antibody-carrying donors. These immunoglobulin solutions, e.g., H-BIG® (Nabi), hep-B-gammagee® (Merck), and HyperHep® (Miles Biologicals), are administered only by intramuscular injection to individuals either as postexposure prophylaxis or as a preventive treatment before an active immunization with hepatitis B vaccine is effective.

The use of human immunoglobulin solutions, for the prevention of either general or specific infections, is called passive immunization. The route of administration of these solutions as indicated on the labels, i.e., for intravenous or intramusclar injection, should be followed strictly in order to avoid anaphylactic shock.

ANIMAL IMMUNOGLOBULINS

Anti-thymocyte equine immunoglobulin (horse IgG) is marketed (ATGAM®, Upjohn) for the management of allograft rejection in renal transplant patients. It reduces the circulated T-lymphocytes and produces a suppressive effect in both cell- and humoral-mediated immunities. This immunoglobulin is usually given by IV infusion, and concomitantly with other immune suppressive drugs.

Anaphylaxis, although uncommon, is the most serious reaction that could occur with animal immunoglobulin therapy. Infusion should be stopped immediately if anaphylaxis occurs and the specific animal immunoglobulins should never be used again on the patient. To avoid this problem, it is recommended that patients should be skin-tested with the specific animal immunoglobulin such as horse immunoglobulin ATGAM® before the first treatment. Other reactions such as chills, fever, itching and erythema, are usually less serious and can be controlled by antihistamines or corticosteroids.

MONOCLONAL ANTIBODIES

Mouse monoclonal anti-CD3 antibodies, e.g., OKT3® from Ortho Biologicals, are used clinically to remove cytotoxic T cells which are responsible for the rejection of graft in kidney transplantation. The treatment of OKT3® can reverse 94% of the rejection, compared to only 75% with conventional immunosuppressive treatment such as steroid therapy. Anti-T cell monoclonal antibodies are also used as an *ex vivo* treatment in bone marrow transplantations. In the cases of T cell leukemia or lymphomas, anti-T cell monoclonal antibodies can be used to purge the bone marrow to remove tumor cells in autologous transplantation. In heterologous transplantations, anti-T cell monoclonal antibodies can be used to remove matured T cells to avoid graft-versus-host (GVH) disease. The use of monoclonal anti-T cell antibodies in transplantation will be discussed in Chapter 8.

Because monoclonal antibodies available at the present time are mostly obtained from mice, one of the most common reactions in using monoclonal antibodies for the treatment of human diseases is the development of human anti-mouse antibody (HAMA). However, this reaction usually occurs 2 to 3 weeks after the initial treatment. Combination with other immunosuppressors, e.g., cyclophosphamide can either delay or decrease HAMA formation.

Two technologies are currently being developed in order to minimize the problems associated with the formation of HAMA in monoclonal antibody-treated patients. As described in Chapter 3, chimeric antibodies, i.e., half human-half mouse immunoglobulins can be prepared by using recombinant technology. For example, a human–mouse chimeric antibody, 7E3, has been successful developed which binds specifically to platelet glycoprotein (GP IIb/IIIa) receptors and, subsequently, inhibits platelet aggregation. The Fab fragment of 7E3, i.e., Abciximab (ReoPro®, Lilly), is used for the prevention of acute cardiac ischemic complications in patients who are at high risk for abrupt closure of angioplasty-treated coronary blood vessels. The other technology is the modification of mouse immunoglobulin genes in order to convert most immunogenically sensitive regions in mouse immunoglobulin to human-like amino acid sequences. Products from this approach are called "humanized antibodies." Several humanized monoclonal antibodies are currently under clinical trials for both therapeutic and diagnostic applications.

Antibodies as Drug Carriers

As we have discussed above, antibodies are usually not cytotoxic by themselves despite their high affinity and selectivity towards the antigens. Therefore, it is reasonable to assume that antibodies would be more effective as carriers targeted to antigen-bearing cells for other bioactive molecules. In this approach, antibodies serve only as vehicles of other drugs to ensure a selective delivery to the diseased tissues or cells. Generally, bioactive agents with either high systemic toxicity or low target tissue absorption most likely will benefit from an antibody carrier. These bioactive agents can be categorized into three major groups:

Therapeutic Drugs — Chemoimmunotherapy

In very few cases, an antibody and a drug have been shown to be synergistic to each other. For example, the anti-tumor activity of alkylating agents such as chlorambucil may be enhanced if anti-tumor antibody is administered simultaneously. In these cases, an increase of the efficacy of the treatment may be achieved simply by using a mixture of the antibody and the drug.

However, in most cases, simply mixing antibody and drug together is not sufficient for the production of any drug targeting effect. In order to achieve the drug targeting effect, a drug must be conjugated to the antibody molecule by a covalent linkage. Various types of chemical linkages have been used for the conjugation of drug and antibody molecules. Some of the representative chemical linkages are listed in Table 4.3. Generally, the linkage should be stable enough to keep the drug and antibody moieties to-

Linkages	Amino Acid Residue Linked	Drug-Releasing Conditions	Compartments Releasing
Peptide	Lys, Glu, Asp, or using peptide spacers	Peptidases Proteases	Most lysosmes Nonlysosomal proteases
Ester and amide	Glu, Asp, Ser, Thr	Esterases and amidase	Lysosomes and plasma membrane
Disulfide	Cys or disulfide spacers	Reduction	Plasma membrane Endosomes Golgi
pH-sensitive	Acid-sensitive spacers	Acidic pH	Endosomes Lysosomes
Glycoside	Carbohydrate moieties	Glycosidase	Lysosomes
Imine and amine	Carbohydrate Moieties (peroxidation and reduction)	Not cleavable	

Table 4.3. Some representative linkages in antibody conjugate preparation.

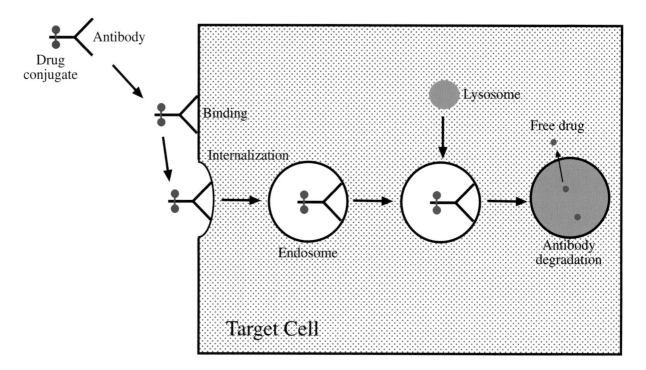

Figure 4.2. Endocytosis of drug–antibody conjugates. Cell surface-bound drug–antibody conjugates can be internalized by the target cells via endocytosis, a vesicular transport process. The internalized drug conjugates will first be delivered to endosomes and later to lysosomes. The conjugates will be digested in lysosomes by lysosomal enzymes. After lysosomal degradation of the antibody, free drug molecules will be released from the conjugate form and reach the action site in the cytoplasm.

gether before reaching the target tissues or cells. However, if a cleavage of the linkage is required for releasing active drug molecules at the target site, the mechanism of cleavage should rely upon the microenvironment of the cellular or the subcellular compartment, e.g., acidification, reduction and proteolysis. The selection of the linkage for the preparation of a drug–antibody conjugate is largely dependent on the nature of the drug, the cellular processing of the antigen, and the mechanism of the drug action. Regarding the site of action, there are two types of drug–antibody conjugates, i.e., conjugates with intracellular action and conjugates with extracellular action.

INTRACELLULAR ACTING ANTIBODY CONJUGATES

For most cancer chemotherapeutic drugs, because their sites of action such as DNA or enzymes are located intracellularly, the surface-bound drug-carrying antibody-antigen complexes must be internalized by the target cell in order to fulfill the ultimate goal of drug delivery. The antibody-antigen complexes are internalized by the cell via endocytosis; a pathway involves formation of intracellular vesicles entrapping membrane-bound macromolecules. The vesicles will be further processed as endosomes and lysosomes, and eventually antibody will be degraded by proteolytic enzymes in lysosomes (Figure 4.2). Two possibilities may prevent the generation of an active drug molecule from its antibody conjugate. First, lysosomes contain many hydrolytic enzymes including not only proteases but also many other enzymes such as glycosidases, nucleases, phosphatase and sulfatase (Table 4.4). In some cases, drug molecules can be degraded and inactivated by one or more of these lysosomal enzymes. This intracellular hydrolysis is particularly formidable for the delivery of peptide or nucleotide drugs via endocytosis. Second, drug-antibody linkage may not be accessible to the enzymatic hydrolysis in the lysosome and, therefore, instead of the original drug molecule, inactive drug-amino acid derivatives may be released from lysosomes (Figure 4.3). Therefore, the desirable site of intracellular releasing as well as the structure-activity relationship of the drug should be considered for designing an appropriate linkage for a specific drug–antibody conjugate.

Proteins and peptides	Polysaccharides	Nucleic acids	Others
Cathepsins (A, B, C, D, E, and L)	α-Glucosidase	Ribonuclease	Phosphatase
Collagenase	β-Glucuronidase	Deoxyribonuclease	Sulfatase
	β-Galactosidase		
	α-Mannosidase		
	β-N-Acetylglucosaminidase		

Table 4.4. Some representative enzymatic degradation in lysosomes.

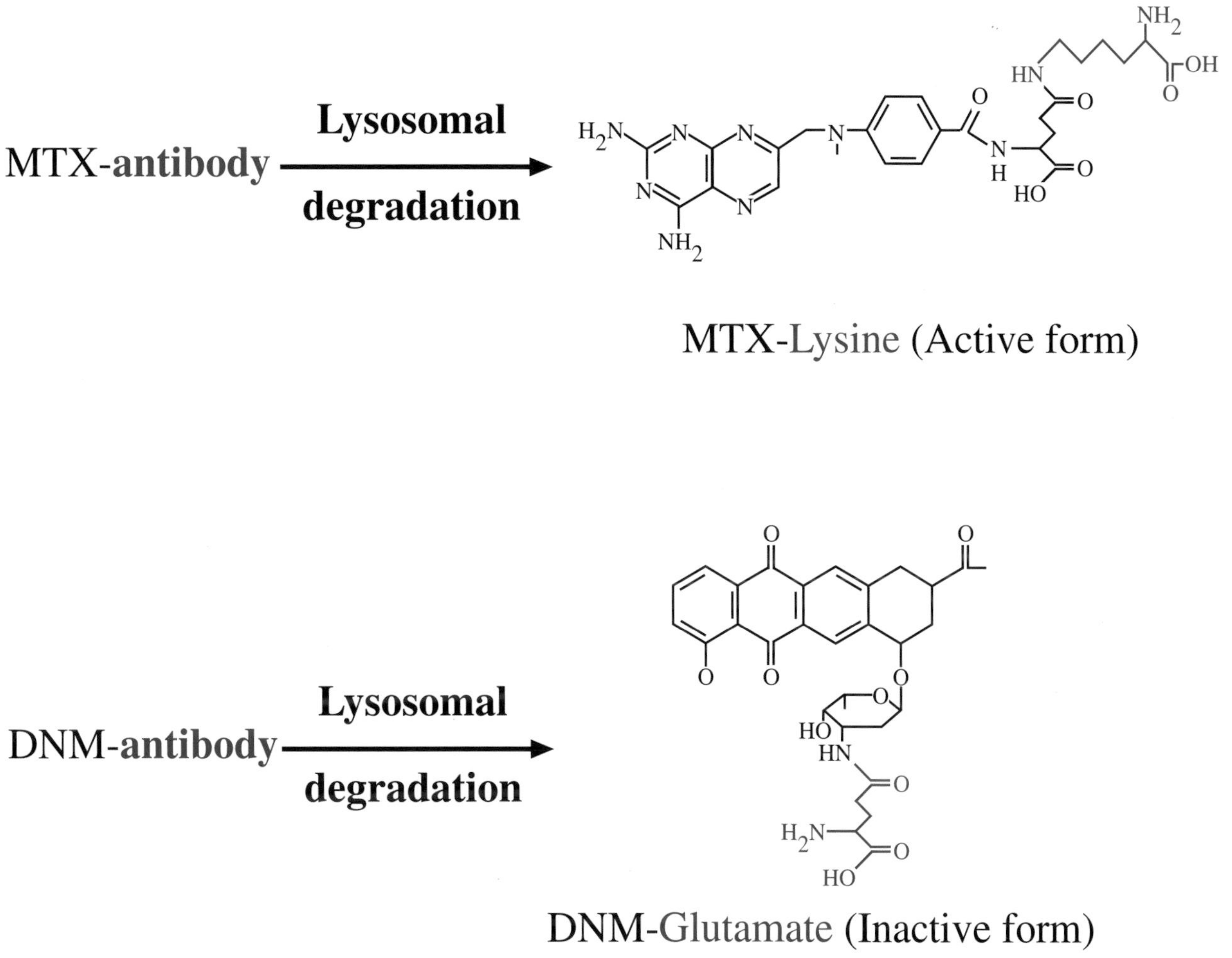

MTX-antibody → Lysosomal degradation → MTX-Lysine (Active form)

DNM-antibody → Lysosomal degradation → DNM-Glutamate (Inactive form)

Figure 4.3. Degradation of drug–antibody conjugates in lysosomes. Methotrexate (MTX) and daunorubicin (DNR) can be directly linked to antibodies. After being internalized by the target cells, lysosomal degradation of these two conjugates will release MTX-lysine and DNR-glutamate, respectively. While MTX-lysine still possesses the anti-folate activity, DNR-glutamate is pharmacologically inactive. Therefore, direct conjugate of MTX and antibody is an active drug conjugate, but that of DNR is not.

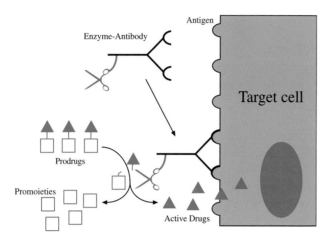

Figure 4.4. Activation of prodrugs by enzyme–antibody conjugates. The prodrug activating enzyme is conjugated to anti-tumor antibody and localized to the tumor sites. When the prodrug is administered later, it can be converted to the active drug only at the surface of the tumor cells, and thus a targeted effect can be achieved. This type of therapy is also called antibody directed enzyme prodrug therapy (ADEPT).

EXTRACELLULAR ACTING ANTIBODY CONJUGATES

Antibody conjugates can have extracellular activity that may result in a targeted drug delivery. One of the extracellular actions is that antibody-carried drugs may exert their effects on the plasma membrane. Alternatively, antibody-carried drugs may be released from the carrier antibody on the surface of the cell which may generate a depot effect on the target tissues.

With the extracellular generation of active drug molecules from antibody conjugates, it is difficult to achieve a high drug concentration at the target site, because the concentration of the free drug is limited by the number of drug molecules conjugated per each antibody, the number of antigenic epitopes on the surface of the target cell, and the releasing rate of the free drug from the conjugate.

However, it has been demonstrated that it is possible to generate active drug molecules at the target site using an enzyme antibody conjugate which can convert an inactive prodrug to an active drug (Figure 4.4). Examples of this approach include the activation of etoposide phosphate by phosphatase-antitumor antibody conjugate, and of N-glutamate derivative of alkylating agents by carboxypeptidase G-antitumor antibody conjugate at the tumor site. Such treatments, known as antibody directed enzyme prodrug therapy (ADEPT), usually require the perfusion of antibody-enzyme conjugate several hours prior to the administration of the prodrug in order to minimize the background enzyme activity due to the presence of unbound antibody-enzyme conjugate in the patient's body.

Toxins — Immunotoxins

As can be seen from Table 4.2, one of the major limitations in using drug–antibody conjugates as targeted carriers is that the amount of drug molecules that can be delivered into the target cell is relatively small and, consequently, a therapeutically efficacious concentration of the drug is difficult to achieve. This limitation, however, could be overcome if a highly potent drug is chosen to prepare the conjugate.

In cancer chemotherapy, drugs usually are chosen based on their cytotoxicity. Generally, there should be a differentiation of toxicity in normal and malignant cells for the selection of a drug in cancer treatment. Highly potent toxic agents are not suitable for cancer chemotherapy due to their systemic toxicity. However, if a highly toxic agent can be linked to an antitumor antibody, the toxic agent will be delivered only to the tumor site but not to normal tissues and a selective killing of tumor cells can be achieved. Such conjugates, which consist of non-therapeutic toxic agents and antibodies, are called immunotoxins. Currently, almost all immunotoxins are prepared from either plant or bacterial protein toxins, because protein toxins usually are among the most toxic agents available (Table 4.5). As shown in Table 4.5, the lethal doses of these toxins are extremely

Type of toxin	Source	LD_{50}*	Mechanism	Mol. W. (Da)
Diphtheria toxin	Corynebacterium diphtheriae	40 ng	Inact. EF-2	62,000
Pseudomonas exotoxin A	Pseudomonas aeruginosa	120 ng	Inact. EF-2	70,000
Abrin	Seeds of Abrus precatorius	13 ng	Inact. rRNA	65,000
Ricin	Seeds of Ricinus communis	65 ng	Inact. rRNA	62,000

* Determined in mice, except for Diphtheria toxin, which was determined in guinea pigs due to the resistance of mice to this toxin.

Table 4.5. Toxins in the preparation of immunotoxins.

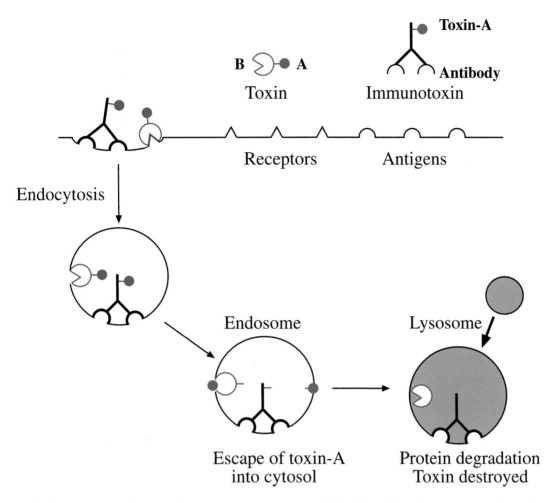

Figure 4.5. Cellular processing of toxins and immunotoxins. Toxins usually bind to cell surface receptors. After endocytosis, the binding domain (B) in the toxin molecule will promote the translocation of the intact live domain (A) from inside the endosome to the cytoplasm where it can exert its cytotoxic effect such as the inhibition of protein synthesis. Immunotoxins generally follow the same pathway as toxins, but it is not clear how the intact active domain can escape from endosome and reach the cytoplasmic target.

low; it has been estimated that the internalization of one active toxin molecule such as ricin is sufficient to kill a mammalian cell. The reason for this extremely high potency of toxicity is that these toxins consist of two polypeptide fragments or subunits. The A-subunit of a toxin possesses enzymatic activity which generally inactivates a cellular pathway in protein biosynthesis. For example, diphtheria toxin A-fragment catalyzes the ADP-ribosylation of elongation factor-2 in ribosomes and ricin A-subunit catalyzes the cleavage of a specifc adenine N-glycosidic bond in ribosomal RNA; both reactions will terminate protein biosynthesis and lead to cell death. The B-subunit of a toxin possesses the binding activity towards specific markers such as glycoproteins or glycolipids on the surface of plasma membranes. In addition to the membrane binding, the B-subunit from most toxins also possesses the activity of transmem-

branous transport of A subunit to ribosomes after the internalization of the toxin molecule by the target cells (Figure 4.5).

Toxins cannot be used as drugs unless they can be altered to target only into the diseased cells such as tumor cells and to abort the binding ability of B-subunits to normal cells. Therefore, immunotoxins prepared from antibody and intact toxin with active B subunit are not suitable for treatment of diseases because the systemic toxicity would be unacceptable for human use. There are several types of immunotoxins with regard to how the conjugates are constructed (Table 4.6). Currently, the most common immunotoxins are prepared from antibody and purified toxin A-subunit linked by a disulfide bond. This type of immunotoxin, although low in systemic toxicity, is not very effective due to the lack of a transmembrane transport

Type	Constituents	Remarks
First generation	Antibody and holotoxin	1. Severe systemic toxicity 2. B-subunit must be blocked or destroyed
Second generation	Antibody and toxin A-subunit	1. Less systemic toxicity 2. Less efficient 3. Used in clinical trials
Third generation	Recombinant chimeric proteins	1. Single chain Fv 2. Selected toxin moieties to increase effectiveness 3. Produced by genetic engineering technology

Table 4.6. Types of Immunotoxin.

mechanism. Recently, it has been found that the transmembrane transport moiety in Pseudomonas exotoxin is distinct from the B-subunit and, therefore, it is possible to construct an immunotoxin from Pseudomonas exotoxin with transmembrane transport activity without the B-subunit. Genetically engineered immunotoxins, also known as chimeric toxins, can be prepared by the fusion of genes from toxin A-subunit and antibody. However, because an antibody molecule consists of four polypeptide chains, which cannot be assembled into an immunoglobulin in non-mammalian cells, recombinant DNA technology has only been successful to produce single-chain Fv-immunotoxin (Chapter 2).

Previously, the use of immunotoxins focused only on the treatment of malignant diseases. However, immunotoxins have been tried recently in the treatment of other types of diseases. Two of the most promising applications are the use of anti-CD8 immunotoxins for the treatment of autoimmune diseases and the use of anti-CD3 immunotoxins as *ex vivo* treatment of bone marrow for the prevention of graft-versus-host disease in bone marrow transplantations (Chapter 8).

Radionuclides — Radioimmunotherapy

Antibodies can carry radioactive nuclides for targeted delivery to specific antigen-bearing tissues or cells. This immuno-localization technique can be applied for the diagnosis of various diseases. However, if a lethal dose of radiation is used, the radioactive antibody can kill the antigen-bearing cells. Clinically, radioimmunotherapy has been demonstrated effective for the treatment of several types of cancers, including liver cancer and lymphomas.

The selection of a suitable radionuclide is critical for the success of radioimmunotherapy. An ideal radionuclide to be carried by antibodies should have an optimal half-life of decay, i.e., not too short to be practical for use and not too

long to be safe for the patient. The radiation emitted from the radionuclide, in contrast to radioimmunodetection, should consist of little or no gamma ray because gamma radiation has a very high penetration ability and can damage normal tissues distant from the target site. Therefore, alpha and beta radiations are preferred for radioimmunotherapy. However, for most alpha emitting radionuclides the half-lives are too short. On the other hand, for most beta radionuclides not only are the half-lives too long but also the energy and tissue penetration are too low to kill mammalian cells. In addition, methods in preparation of antibody conjugates may also limit the selection of radionuclide for radioimmunotherapy. Currently, the best choice of the radionuclide is ^{90}Y which is a pure beta-emitter, and has a half-life of 64 hours and an emission energy of 2.27 MeV. ^{131}I, on the other hand, emits a small fraction of gamma radiation, but has been used very often in radioimmunotherapy due to the desirable half-life (8 days), the high energy of the beta emission (about 1 MeV), and most importantly, the convenience in coupling to antibody by standard protein iodination procedures. However, the occurrence of dehalogenation reaction in normal tissues can potentially remove ^{131}I from the antibody molecule and cause unwanted side effects including the inhibition of thyroid function.

Comparison of Different Agents in Antibody-Mediated Drug Delivery

We have discussed in this chapter three types of agents that can be delivered to a target site via an antibody-mediated delivery system. The question is which one of the three types of antibody conjugates is most effective in therapeutic uses. Unfortunately, none of them has a clear advantage over the others; therefore, the choice of the agent is largely dependent on the disease and the availability of the antibody conjugate. However, there are several distinct

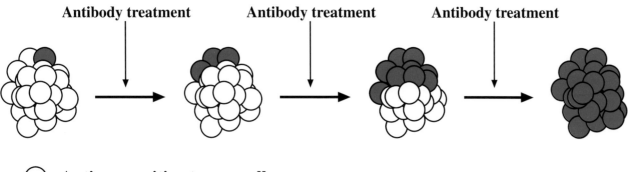

Antibody treatment   **Antibody treatment**   **Antibody treatment**

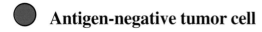

○ **Antigen-positive tumor cell**

● **Antigen-negative tumor cell**

Figure 4.6. Antigen heterogeneity in antibody-mediated cancer treatment. The heterogeneity of tumor antigens even within a single tumor mass makes antibody-mediated cancer treatment difficult to kill all tumor cells. As shown in this figure, selective growth of antigen-negative tumor cells may occur during the treatment. To overcome this problem, it is recommended using either radioimmunotherapy which can kill cells within a radiation range, or using antibody cocktails which consist of a mixture of antibodies to all possible antigens of the specific type of tumor.

features among these three types of agents which should be considered when a choice has to be made.

(a) The effective dose of the agent: As we have already discussed, one of the limiting factors for the therapeutic drug–antibody conjugates is that the number of drug molecules per antibody is very small, i.e., less than 10 per IgG. In addition, the molecular weight of an antibody, i.e., a minimum of 150 kDa for IgG, is 100 to 1,000-fold larger than that of a conventional therapeutic drug. Therefore, in order to achieve a therapeutic effective dose, a very high concentration of the antibody may be needed to carry an effective amount of drug molecules. In this regard, a toxin clearly has the advantage over a therapeutic drug due to the extremely high potency (Table 4.5). Recent development on the prodrug enzyme–antibody conjugates may also overcome the problem of the low concentration of active drugs carried by antibody. Because pharmacokinetic properties and side effects of therapeutic drugs are well-established and are familiar to clinicians, drug–antibody and prodrug enzyme–antibody conjugates are still being considered despite many shortcomings associated with their applications.

(b) The internalization of membrane-bound antibody complexes: In drug–antibody conjugates and immunotoxins, the therapeutic effect is dependent on the endocytosis of the surface antigen-bound antibody conjugates. An effective endocytosis includes not only the internalization of the conjugate, but also the intracellular release of active agents. This process is a limiting factor for antibody-mediated delivery of therapeutic drug and toxin. Prodrug enzyme–antibody conjugates can avoid this problem, but the transport of active drug across plasma membrane could be a limiting factor. On the other hand, radionuclides do not require the internalization of conjugates for the cytotoxicity, and this is a clear advantage of radioimmunotherapy over chemoimmunotherapy.

(c) The heterogeneity of antigens on target cells: One of the most serious problems in using antibodies as drugs or drug carriers is that there may not be a universal antigen on the surface of all diseased cells from an individual patient. This is a very likely problem in cancer treatment because it has been shown that antigen heterogeneity exists even within a single solid tumor mass. Therefore, treatment with drug or toxin conjugates of a specific antibody may selectively promote the growth of antigen-negative tumor cells (Figure 4.6). In order to avoid incomplete cell killing, mixtures of antibodies, or antibody cocktails, against various antigens from a single type of cancer cells should be used as the carrier of drugs or toxins. This problem of antigen heterogeneity can also be overcome if a radionuclide is used instead of drugs or toxins. Radionuclides used in radioimmunotherapy have a tissue penetration distance larger than the diameter of a single cell and thus the binding of radioactive antibody to an antigen-positive cell in a solid tumor will kill several cells in its proximity. Consequently, antigen-negative cells coexisting with antigen-positive cells within a solid tumor will also be killed. However, this non-specific cytotoxicity on antigen-negative cells, especially on radioactive antibody encountered cells other than in the target tissue, can cause unwanted side-effects in patients with radio-immunotherapeutic treatments.

Safety and Efficacy of Antibodies in Therapeutic Applications

During the last several years, increasing number of antibodies, especially monoclonal antibodies, have become available as therapeutic drugs for the treatment of human diseases. There are even a larger number of antibodies and antibody derivatives such as immunotoxins currently under clinical trials and their approval can be anticipated in the very near future. Antibodies are different from conventional drugs, and, therefore, different criteria must be imposed when they are evaluated for safety and efficacy in therapeutic applications.

Immunoglobulins isolated from human serum, like other blood products, must be screened carefully for any potential pathogens. This is particularly important for viral contamination which may lead to serious infections such as hepatitis and AIDS. Monoclonal antibodies produced by hybridoma technology must also be screened carefully for any contaminated materials especially virus before administered to patients. Although no incident has yet been reported, viral contamination, which could be derived from hybridomas themselves or from hybridoma-carrying animals for the production of monoclonal antibodies, may cause unwanted side effects or even diseases.

Another safety requirement for therapeutic application of antibodies is the crossreactivity towards antigens on normal cells. The crossreactivity of an antibody to normal tissues can cause unpredictable side effects in patients, especially when a cytotoxic antibody or antibody conjugate is administered. It is important to realize that different batches of antibody against an identical antigen may possess different crossreactivity to other antigenic structures.

The effective dosage of an antibody is difficult to select because the criteria for the efficacy and side effects are different from those used in conventional drugs. Furthermore, the effect of an antibody is dependent on the individual patient's condition, which includes many diverse factors such as the blood level of free antigen molecule, the previous and current treatment with chemotherapeutic drugs, the immune competency and sensitivity, and the accessibility of the diseased cells.

One of the most commonly occurring side effects of antibodies either as drugs or drug carriers is the development of hypersensitivity in patients. For example, transplant patients after receiving horse anti-thymocyte antiserum as an immunosuppressor may develop hypersensitivity towards horse serum proteins. Similarly, patients receiving mouse monoclonal antibody may develop human anti-mouse antibody (HAMA) which can either abolish the therapeutic effect of the antibody or elicit allergic reactions. Therefore, anaphylactic reactions should be monitored carefully in patients who are receiving multiple doses of same type of antibody in a period of two weeks or longer. Until biotechnology can produce clinically desirable human or humanized monoclonal antibodies, hypersensitivity will always be a concern for the use of antibodies as drugs or drug carriers. ■

References

- **Bruland OS.** (1995). Cancer therapy with radiolabled antibodies. An overview. *Acta Oncol*, **34**, 1085–1094
- **Deonarain MP, Epenetos AA.** (1994). Targeting enzymes for cancer therapy: Old enzymes in new roles. *Br J Cancer*, **70**, 786–794
- **Ghetie MA, Vitetta ES.** (1994). Recent developments in immunotoxin therapy. *Curr Opin Immunol*, **6**, 707–714
- **Harrington KJ, Epenetos AA.** (1995). Recent developments in radioimmunotherapy. *Clin Oncol*, **6**, 391–398
- **Knox SJ.** (1995). Overview of studies on experimental radioimmunotherapy. *Cancer Res*, **55** (23 Suppl), 5832s–5836s
- **Melton RG, Sherwood RF.** (1996). Antibody-enzyme conjugates for cancer therapy. *J Natl Cancer Inst*, **88**, 153–165
- **Pastan IH, Pai LH, Brinkmann U, Fitzgerald DJ.** (1995). Recombinant toxins: new therapeutic agents for cancer. *Ann NY Acad Sci*, **758**, 345–354
- **Pietersz GA, Krauer K.** (1994). Antibody-targeted drugs for the therapy of cancer. *J Drug Targeting*, **2**, 183–215
- **Reilly RM, Sandhu J, Alvarez-Diez TM, Gallinger S, Kirsh J, Stern H.** (1995). Problems of delivery of monoclonal antibodies. Pharmaceutical and pharmacokinetic solutions. *Clin Pharmacokinet*, **28**, 126–142

Case Studies with Self-Assessment Questions

Case 1

B3, a murine monoclonal antibody, recognizes a carbohydrate antigen (Le^y) present on many human solid tumors. This monoclonal antibody was used to prepare an immunotoxin, LMB-1, by chemically linking it to a genetically engineered form of Pseudomonas exotoxin, PE38. Phase I study of LMB-1 was carried out in the National Cancer Institute, USA, on 38 patients with advanced solid tumors. Patients with either colorectal, esophageal, or breast cancer, who had failed conventional therapy and whose tumors expressed the Le^y antigen, were included in this study. The maximum tolerated dose of LMB-1 is 75 mg/kg given intravenously three times every other day. With this dosage, which is about 1/10 of that used for the treatment of human tumor-bearing nude mice, the only major side effect of LMB-1 was the vascular leak syndrome manifested by hypoalbuminemia, fluid retention, and hypotension.

Three weeks after the treatment, all patients developed antibody titers against PE38, where 33/38 had antibody titers against monoclonal antibody B3. Objective antitumor activity was observed in 5 patients and complete remission was observed in only one patient. Currently, a genetic engineered chimeric toxin, LMB-7, which consists of a single-chain B3(sFv) fused with PE-38, is used to replace LMB-1 for further clinical trials.

Question 1:   *Why did only 5 out of 38 patients show positive response to treatment with LMB-1, even though all of the tumors were Le^y -positive?*

Question 2:   *What is the most likely cause of the vascular leak syndrome?*

Question 3:   *What are the possible improvements that may increase the efficacy of LMB-1 treatment?*

Question 4:   *Do you think that the host antibody formation against LMB-1 is a major problem in the immunotoxin therapy?*

Question 5:   *What are advantages of using chimeric toxin LMB-7, instead of toxin-antibody conjugate LMB-1, in cancer therapy?*

Answer 1:   Several factors may contribute to the low response rate of the therapy. First, not all solid tumors are equally accessible to the administered immunotoxin molecules. The location, size, antigen heterogeneity, and vascularity can determine the amount of immunotoxin actually targeted to the tumor cells. Secondly, the doses administered may not be optimum for the treatment. As noticed in this case, the doses used were significantly lower than those used in animal experiments; therefore, it is difficult to extrapolate therapeutic efficacy from experimental animals to humans. However, the systemic toxicity of the immunotoxin at higher doses is a serious concern, which makes it difficult to dose-escalate to optimize therapy. Thirdly, patients with cancer at advanced stages were selected for this phase I clinical trial. Since all of them had failed previously in conventional chemotherapy, some of the mechanisms in resistance to chemotherapeutic drugs may have cross-activity to the immunotoxins.

Answer 2:   The vascular leak syndrome may be due to the presence of small number of Le^y antigen on the surface of endothelial cells. It may be also due to non-specific binding of LMB-1 on the surface of endothelial cells such as charge or hydrophobic interaction.

Answer 3:   Increasing dosage may improve the efficacy of immunotoxins; however, the systemic toxicity should be considered seriously. To overcome the problem of antigen-heterogeneity, immunotoxins are prepared from antibody-cocktails, i.e., a mixture of antibodies against different antigen epitopes on the tumor cell surface. Another possible approach is to use enhancers, such as verapamil and monensin, to increase the efficacy of immunotoxins. However, this approach is still an experimental therapy.

Answer 4: Host antibody formation, such as HAMA in this case, is a problem for the use of therapeutic monoclonal antibodies. It is likely that the anti-LMB-1 antibody in the patients may neutralize and prevent the binding of the immunotoxin to tumor antigens. However, as indicated in this case, positive responses were observed in five patients even though antibody was detected in all patients after treatment. Therefore, the host antibody against the immunotoxin may not completely abolish the tumor targeting effect.

Answer 5: The molecular size of the chimeric toxin, LMB-7, is smaller than that of the conjugate toxin, LMB-1. Therefore, LMB-7 may be more permeable to the vascular endothelium and more accessible to the tumor mass. It also may be less antigenic than LMB-1 molecule. In addition, LMB-7 is prepared by using genetic engineering technology which should be more practical than the chemical preparation method for LMB-1 regarding purity, quantity, costs, etc.

Case 2

Stage-specific embryonic antigen-1 (SSEA-1) is a tumor-associated antigen, which can be detected on the surface of teratocarcinoma cells. The other tissue, which contains a high level of SSEA-1, is the kidney. A murine IgM monoclonal antibody directed SSEA-1 (anti-SSEA-1) was produced using hybridoma technology. When the radiolabeled (radioactive iodine-131) anti-SSEA-1 was injected intravenously into teratocarcinoma-bearing mice, radioactivity was predominantly detected at the site of the tumor one day after administration.

Question 1: *Explain why the radiolabeled anti-SSEA-1 does not localize in the kidneys even though SSEA-1 antigen can be detected in kidney tissue.*

Question 2: *Do you expect that the solid tumor of teratocarcinoma will be eliminated by the anti-SSEA-1 treatment?*

Question 3: *Does the selective tumor localization of anti-SSEA-1 warrant that this monoclonal antibody is effective for targeted delivery of anti-cancer agents to teratocarcinoma cells?*

Question 4: *What will be your concerns with the development of anti-SSEA-1 as drug carrier for the treatment of human teratocarcinoma patients?*

Answer 1: One of the reasons that anti-SSEA-1 monoclonal antibody does not localize in the kidneys is that the antigens in kidney tissue may not be accessible to the circulating antibody in the blood. It is also possible that the retention of antibody in the tumor is higher than that in the kidneys.

Answer 2: Most likely not. Antibodies usually are not cytotoxic to the antigen-bearing cells.

Answer 3: It is difficult to evaluate by the information presented in this case. Tumor imaging is dependent on the target/non-target ratio of the antibody concentrations. However, for the targeted delivery of chemotherapeutic drugs, the absolute amount of drugs that is delivered into the tumor mass is critical.

Answer 4: The permeability of anti-SSEA-1, an IgM antibody, across the vascular wall to reach the tumor cells is one of the concerns because it may determine whether there will be enough drug molecules to be delivered to the tumor cells or not. In addition, many factors such as the internalization and the modulation of SSEA-1 on the surface of teratocarcinoma cells are unknown.

5 Hypersensitivity and Drug Allergy

The immune system is a destructive organization in the human body which constantly destroys invading microorganisms from the environment using mechanisms such as complement fixation, ADCC, cytotoxic T cells, and reactions involving many other cytotoxic factors. Therefore, it is not surprising that some of the immune reactions may actually damage host tissues due to an overresponse to certain antigens; this undesirable response of the immune system to the specific antigen, also known as allergen, is allergy. The subsequent immunological reaction after the exposure to the allergen is hypersensitivity; but, generally the terms allergy and hypersensitivity are used interchangeably in many occasions. Hypersensitivity can be considered as a result of the "double-edged sword" effect of the immune system and some of the hypersensitive responses possibly also play positive roles in the self-defense process. However, many reactions in hypersensitivity appear to have no apparent beneficial effect on the human body. It is very likely that during the evolution of the immune system, the infectious agents have changed drastically in the environment and, therefore, the functions of these immune reactions have become obsolete. For example, it is suggested that the anaphylactic response from allergic reaction is a critical mechanism for the defense against certain types of parasitic infections which may be uncommon today. In fact, it has been demonstrated that the production of IgE against parasites such as in schistosomiasis is an important event in humans who have acquired a high resistance to the parasitic infection.

There are four different types of hypersensitivity, namely types I, II, III, and IV (Figure 5.1); each type of hypersensitivity carries a unique mechanism that can cause tissue damage (Table 5.1).

Type I Hypersensitivity

Type I hypersensitivity, also known as the immediate type hypersensitivity, is the most common form of the allergic reaction. It may result in an uncomfortable but harmless condition, such as hay fever or spring fever, or a life-threatening situation, such as anaphylactic reasponse to allergens or drugs. In both cases, the responses occur shortly after the exposure of an antigen to the body which had previously been sensitized to that specific antigen. The initiation stage of the allergic reaction begins with the contact of a multivalent antigen, either a natural pollent or a synthetic drug molecule, to IgE-class antibodies which

Type	Type I	Type II	Type III	Type IV
Synonym	Anaphylatic	Cytotoxic	Immune Complex	Delay-type
Antibody	IgE	IgG and IgM	IgG and other	None
Antigen	Atopic	Cell membrane-associated	Soluble	Tissue-associated
Target cell	Mast cells	Erythrocytes, etc.	Endothelium, etc.	Macrophages
Mediators	Histamines, leukotrienes, etc.	Complements	Complements, vasodilators, etc.	Interleukins
Target Tissues	Smooth muscle	Blood, etc.	Kidneys, etc.	Varies
Example	Hay fever, Anaphylaxis	Blood transfusion reaction	Serum sickness	Contact dermatitis

Table 5.1. Classification of hypersensitivities.

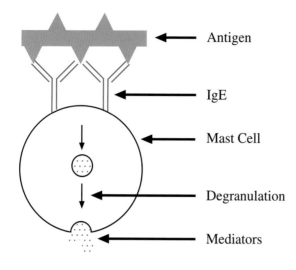

Type I Hypersensitivity

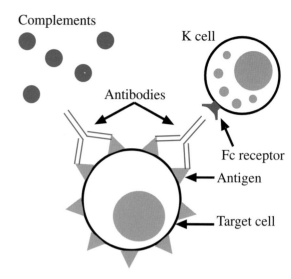

Type II Hypersensitivity

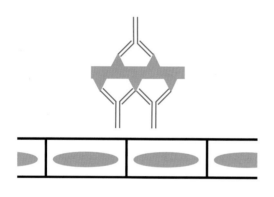

Type III Hypersensitivity

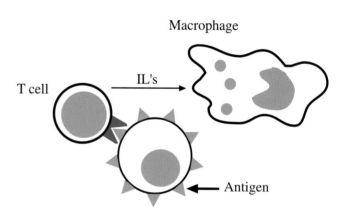

Type IV Hypersensitivity

Figure 5.1. The four different types of hypersensitivity. Type I hypersensitivity is mediated by the cross-reaction of mast cell surface-bound IgE molecules by polyvalent antigens such as pollens. Such a binding will promote the degranulation and, subsequently, the release of mediators by the mast cell. Type II hypersensitivity is initiated when antibodies bind to antigen-bearing or -bound target cells. A target cell can be killed by either k cell-mediated cytotoxicity (IgG antibodies) or complement-mediated cytotoxicity (IgG or IgM). Type III hypersensitivity involves the formation of antibody–antigen complexes which mostly are IgG antibody. When attached to tissues such as endothelium from the blood, the immune complexes can attract granulocytes or complement factors and subsequently damage the tissue. Type IV hypersensitivity does not involve antibodies. This type hypersensitivity is initiated by the contact of T lymphocytes with their primed antigens and subsequently the release of interleukins from the T lymphocytes will elicit macrophages into an inflammatory state. Details of each type of hypersensitivity are described in this chapter.

are bound to mast cell surface via Fc$_\varepsilon$-receptors — receptors selectively bind the Fc-region of an IgE immunoglobulin molecule. This binding causes the crosslinking of mast cell surface IgE antibodies via antigens, increases the influx of calcium ions, and, subsequently, triggers the degranulation of mediator-containing granules. Degranulation occurs when an intracellular granule fuses with the plasma membrane and releases the contained mediators into the extracellular

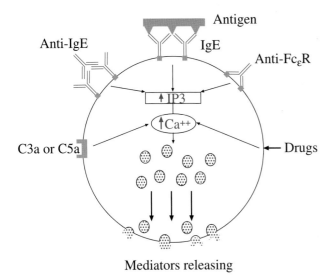

Antigen

Anti-IgE   IgE

Anti-FcεR

↑IP3

↑Ca++

C3a or C5a   Drugs

Mediators releasing

Figure 5.2. The degranulation of mast cells. The crosslinking of IgE molecules which are bound to the Fcε receptors (FcεR) on the surface of mast cells can increase the inositol-3–phosphate (IP3) due to the activation of phospholipases. IP3, in turn, can increase calcium ion influx which triggers the movement of intracellular secretory granules toward the plasma membrane and, subsequently, the fusion of granular membrane with the plasma membrane causes the release of intragranular mediators to the outside of the mast cell. Several other events can mimic the action of antigen-IgE interaction such as the crosslinking of mast cell-surface IgE by using anti-IgE antibodies or the crosslinking of FcεR by using anti-FcεR antibodies. Other endogenous factors such as C3a and C5a, or exogenous factors such as several types of drug also cause the influx of calcium ions and, therefore, the degranulation of mast cells.

fluid (Figure 5.2). Several other conditions besides the antigen-IgE interaction can also trigger the degranulation in mast cells and, therefore, can cause type I hypersensitivity. Two of the most common causes other than antigen-IgE interaction are (a) drug-induced degranulation and (b) degranulation induced by endogenous factors.

Drug Induced Mast Cell Degranulation

Drug molecules may stimulate mast cell degranulation without involving IgE and Fcε-receptors on the cell surface. Ionophores, which can increase the influx of calcium ions, may mimic antigen-IgE interactions and subsequently release allergic mediators from mast cells. Some of the venoms such as mellitin from bee stings can interact with mast cells and produce allergy-like reactions. Similarly, anti-IgE or anti-Fcε-receptor antibodies can also mimic allergic reactions by virtue of their capabilities to cross-link mast cell surface IgE molecules or Fcε-receptors.

Many drugs can produce allergy-like reactions possibly due to their effects on the degranulation in mast cells. Narcotic drugs, including morphine and codeine, are known to cause allergy-like reactions. Other drugs that may have similar effects include polymyxin B sulfate, d-tubocurarine iodide, and synthetic ACTH. Iodinated organic compounds used as contrast media in diagnostic imaging procedures may also induce mast cell degranulation (Table 5.2). However, the number of drugs that can induce mast cell degranulation is relatively small and, therefore, it is not a major cause of drug allergy. Since this reaction is not mediated by an immune response to the drugs, it is referred to as pseudo-allergy.

Endogenous Factors Induced Mast Cell Degranulation

As we have already discussed in Chapter 2, anaphylatoxins, i.e., C3a and C5a, generated from complement reactions can induce the degranulation in mast cells. However, C3a and C5a can have effects on other types of cells such as monocytes and granulocytes.

Mediators in Type I Hypersensitivity

Mediators released from mast cells upon antigen or drug stimulation can be classified into two different categories: the preformed mediators and the newly synthesized mediators (Table 5.3).

	Fcε receptor-mediated	Drug-mediated	Complement-mediated
Factors	IgE- or Fcε receptor-crossing agents	Small molecules	Complement fragments
Examples	Plant pollens, lectins, anti-IgE or anti-Fcε receptor antibodies	Mellitin, ATCH, codeine, morphine, anesthetics, diatrizoate, etc.	C3a and C5a

Table 5.2. Factors triggering the degranulation of mast cells.

Type of mediators	Mediator	Major activity	Antagonist
Preformed	Histamine	Contraction of smooth muscle	Antihistamines
	Heparin	Anticoagulant	Protamines
	Proteases	Activation of kinins and complements	Protease inhibitors
	Eosinophil chemotactic factor of anaphylaxis (ECF-A)	Chemotaxis	Unknown
Newly-synthesized	Prostaglandins	Inhibit degranulation	Indomethacin and aspirin
	Leukotrienes	Contraction of smooth	Indomethacin
	Thromboxanes	Platelet aggregation	Indomethacin
	Platelet activating activating factor (PAF)	Platelet aggregation	Phospholipase

Table 5.3. Mediators of Type I hypersensitivity.

THE PREFORMED MEDIATORS

Preformed mediators are stored in granules inside mast cells. Upon responding to outside stimulations such as antigen-IgE interaction the granules will fuse with the plasma membrane and the contents will be released by a process which is similar to that of exocytosis in secretory cells. The most important mediator preformed in the granules is histamine which is stored in the granules as a complex of an anionic macromolecule, heparin. After being released, histamine will bind to either H1 or H2 receptors on the surface of a variety of cells. Binding to receptors on the surface of endothelial cells will loosen the tight junction and increase vascular permeability, an effect that may cause tissue edema and a drop in blood pressure. On the other hand, binding to the receptors on the surface of smooth muscle cells will cause constriction, an effect that may cause difficulty in breathing due to the constriction of the bronchi in the lungs. Both the edema and the asphyxiation are symptoms of anaphylaxis and are potentially fatal. In addition to the anaphylactic effects, binding of H_2 receptors also causes the release of acid from stomach mucosa; therefore, H_2-antagonists have been used as drugs for the treatment of stomach ulcer. In some animal systems, serotonin is the major, small molecular mediator released from mast cells in anaphylactic reactions.

There are several other components pre-exising in the granules that are released from mast cells in the type I hypersensitivity. Heparin, in addition to the formation of histamine complexes in the storage form, can have antico-agulant activity as well as binding to complement factors when released from mast cells. Several proteases are also present in the granules of mast cells. These enzymes are involved indirectly in the anaphylactic reaction because they can act on many serum proteins to generate active fragments such as C3a and C5a from complement factors and bradykinin, a vasodilating peptide, from α_2-globulin.

NEWLY SYNTHESIZED MEDIATORS

Calcium ion influx that triggers the degranulation of mast cells can also activate phospholipase A_2, an enzyme that releases arachidonic acid from phospholipids in plasma membranes. The released arachidonic acid can be further oxidized by the enzyme lipooxygenase to form leukotriene A. Leukotriene A can be converted to stable leukotrienes C, D and E. Arachidonic acid can also be oxidized by the enzyme cyclooxygenase to form prostaglandins and thromboxanes. Many of these arachidonic acid derivatives cause bronchial muscle contraction and vasodilation, and some of them may result in activity of chemotaxis or platelet aggregation, as well; therefore, they are usually referred to as slow-reacting substances of anaphylaxis (SRS-A).

During the release of arachidonic acid from phospholipids by phospholipase A_2, a group of phosphorylcholine derivatives is also generated. These compounds can cause platelet and neutrophil aggregation, and are known as platelet activating factors (PAF). PAF can also increase vascular permeability and, possibly, the smooth muscle contraction.

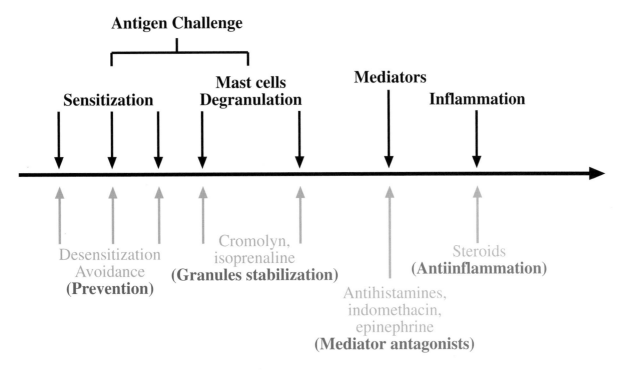

Figure 5.3. Different stages in type I hypersensitivity and their treatments. The horizontal arrow indicates the progress of the time. The black arrows indicate the stages of hypersensitivity development. The blue arrows indicate the prevention or treatment at various stages.

ANAPHYLAXIS

Type I hypersensitivity could result in anaphylaxis depending on the type, the dose and the biodistribution of allergens. Systemic anaphylaxis occurs after the secondary exposure to the allergen which is distributed rapidly through the whole body. Systemic anaphylaxis can be fatal due to asphyxiation caused by the contraction of the smooth muscle of the bronchi and edema in the lungs.

TYPES OF ALLERGY

Atopic allergy, hypersensitivity to extrinsic antigens, usually occurs in either the respiratory or the digestive system. Common allergens in respiratory atopic allergy are pollens of plants, spores of fungi, and mites and their fecal pellets in dust. Symptoms of this type of allergy include many local anaphylactic reactions such as sneezing, nasal discharge, weeping red eyes, and swollen mucosa. They are a nuisance but generally not life-threatening. However, atopic allergy in the respiratory system can develop into asthma. Asthma is characterized by the obstruction of the respiratory airway as a consequence of smooth muscle contraction, bronchial edema, and mucus hypersecretion. Furthermore, mast cell-released chemotactic factors attract neutrophils and macrophages and may lead to the chronic inflammatory response associated with asthmatic symptoms.

Food allergy usually happens immediately following the intake of specific foods. The symptoms of food allergy include swollen lips and inside of the mouth, intestinal cramping, nausea, and diarrhea. In some cases, urticaria, or hives, may result from antigens entering specific areas of the skin and causing local vasodilation and edema in certain parts of the body.

Control of Type I Hypersensitivity

The control of type I hypersensitivity is dependent on the stage of the allergic reaction (Figure 5.3). If an allergen can be identified, the most effective method for the intervention of the allergy is to avoid the source of the antigen such as specific plants or animals. Alternatively, desensitization may be effective for individuals with severe allergic reactions. The desensitization process is usually carried out by intramuscularly administering a series of gradually increasing doses of the allergen to the individual during a period of months. This process is intended to generate IgG antibodies against the allergen that will prevent its binding to the mast cell-associated IgE antibodies. However, the exact mechanism of desensitization is still not fully understood.

The elicitation of anaphylaxis during the desensitization process is a serious concern for this treatment. Therefore, desensitization usually is not the first choice for the treatment of allergy or asthma, and is used only when there is no other therapeutic options.

Once the allergen has reached the mast cells, the release of mediators such as histamine and leukotrienes can be prevented by cromolyn, which stabilizes mast cells against degranulation. Other types of drugs such as theophylline and caffeine, although they act primarily as bronchodilators, can also increase the intracellular concentration of cAMP and, in turn, stabilize mast cell granules.

Allergy treatments usually are sought only after the symptoms have appeared, a stage at which the degranulation of mast cells has already occurred. Therefore, antihistamines, the antagonists of histamine, are used most frequently for the treatment of allergic symptoms. Antihistamines may be effective in competing with histamine-receptor binding but not in displacing receptor-bound histamine; consequently, antihistamines are not always useful for the treatment of allergic symptoms when histamine has already reached endothelial or smooth muscle cells. In addition, other mediators such as leukotrienes are also responsible for anaphylactic reactions which cannot be prevented by antihistamines. To decrease the formation of leukotrienes, prostaglandins, and thromboxanes inhibitors for the arachidonic acid metabolizing enzymes such as indomethacin and aspirin can be used.

The action of histamine and other mediators can be reversed by administering the adrenergic drugs, which are generally sympathomimetic amines and can induce bronchodilation and smooth muscle relaxation. In addition, these drugs can also stabilize mast cells from degranulation. Therefore, adrenergic drugs such as epinephrine are commonly used for the treatment of relatively serious anaphylactic reactions. For the late stage of allergic reaction, many inflammatory factors may participate. In these cases, anti-inflammation drugs such as steroids may be required for the treatment.

Type I Hypersensitivity in Drug Allergy

Drug-induced anaphylaxis is uncommon but a serious problem in drug allergic reaction because it is life-threatening. This type of drug reaction is becoming increasingly important because many protein drugs such as monoclonal antibodies and cytokines produced by hybridoma and recombinant DNA technologies are now commercially available as therapeutic agents. Repeated intravenous administration of proteins from non-human or modified human origins may induce immunological responses and, if involving IgE formation, anaphylaxis.

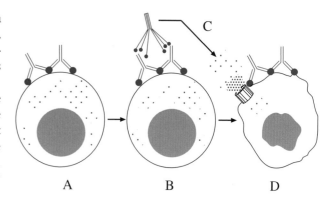

Figure 5.4. Mechanism of complement-mediated cytotoxicity in type II hypersensitivity. Type II hypersensitivity is initiated when antibodies, either IgG or IgM, bind to antigens on the surface of a target cell such as red blood cell (A). The cross-binding of C1 complement factor to two adjacent antibodies at Fc regions (B) will initiate the cascade reaction (C) as described in Chapter 5, and cytolysis occurs when membrane-attack complexes (MAC) are formed (D).

Small molecular drugs may also be implicated in anaphylactic reactions. In several cases, such as penicillin, drug molecules or metabolites may conjugate to serum proteins and act as haptens to elicit immunologic responses. Other drugs such as anesthetics, when administered intravenously, may also produce anaphylactic reactions possibly mediated by a non-immunologic mechanism, i.e., a direct interaction with mast cells.

Type II Hypersensitivity

Type II hypersensitivity, also known as cytotoxic hypersensitivity, is caused by the antibody-mediated cytotoxicity towards antigen-positive cells. Two general mechanisms can account for the antibody-mediated killing of antigen-bearing cells, i.e., complement-mediated cytolysis (CMC) and antibody-dependent cell-mediated cytotoxicity (ADCC). As discussed in Chapter 2, CMC can be carried out by either IgG or IgM immunoglobulins, but ADCC is limited only to IgG class antibody.

The mechanisms involved in complement-mediated cytotoxicity (Figure 5.4) have already been discussed in Chapter 2. Both IgM and IgG can initiate a complement reaction, but IgM is more effective in causing agglutination of antigen-bearing cells such as erythrocytes. Complement-mediated type II hypersensitivity may indirectly induce type I hypersensitivity via the formation of C3a and C5a anaphylatoxins.

Blood group	Erythrocyte antigen	Genotype	Serum Antibody
A	A	AA or AO	Anti-B
B	B	BB or BO	Anti-A
AB	A and B	AB	None
O	None	OO	Anti-A and anti-B

Table 5.4. Human ABO blood groups and serum antibodies.

The mechanism involved in ADCC has been discussed in Chapter 4. ADCC is dependent on not only the isotypes of IgG but also the availability of effector cells such as macrophages and K cells, and is a process observed mostly in *in vitro* models; its exact role in the immunological response to antibody-bound target cells is still uncertain.

The most common type II hypersensitivity in humans is the blood antigen reactions, including the responses towards ABO and Rhesus (Rh) antigens. ABO groups are the most dominant blood antigens in human (Table 5.4). ABO antigens consist of a carbohydrate moiety, substance H, with different modifications. Group A and group B individuals carry an N-acetylgalactosamine- and a galactose-modified substance H, respectively. Group AB individuals carry substance H modified by both N-acetylgalactosamine and galactose, while group O individuals carry non-modified substance H. Consequently, anti-B antigen antibodies are found in the serum of A antigen-carrying individuals, and vice versa. Similarly, both anti-A and anti-B antibodies are found in O group individuals, while neither anti-A nor anti-B is found in group AB individuals. Severe reactions, including fever, chills, hypotension, nausea, vomiting, hemoglobulinemia, hemoglobulinuria, and renal failure, will develop when a recipient of a blood transfusion receives blood from a donor that contains reactive antigens towards the recipient's serum antibodies.

Rhesus antigen is the major cause of hemolytic disease in human newborn (HDNB). HDNB occurs when the anti-fetal erythrocyte antigen IgG immunoglobulins in the mother's blood cross the placenta into the fetal circulation. The IgG antibodies will cause the hemolysis of fetal erythrocytes. Rhesus antigen D (RhD), also known as the Rh factor or Rh_0, is the most common antigen that is responsible for HDNB. An RhD antigen negative, or Rh⁻, mother can be sensitized with RhD antigen during the birth of a RhD antigen positive, or Rh⁺ baby. Anti-Rh⁺ antibodies present in the mother's blood after the birth will affect Rh⁺ fetuses in future pregnancies. HDNB now can be effectively prevented by giving anti-Rh⁺ antibodies to the mother shortly after the first birth of a Rh incompatible baby. Generally, anti-Rh⁺ solutions, such as Rh Gamulin Rh® (Armour), HypRho-D® (Miles Biologicals), and RhoGAM® (Ortho) are administered intramuscularly within 72 hours after the delivery of a full-term infant. The antibodies will bind Rh antigens on the blood cells of the newborn which are present in the mother's circulation due to fetomaternal hemorrhage during the delivery. Consequently, the immune response of the mother to form her own anti-Rh⁺ antibodies is prevented. Delaying the administration after 72 hours will reduce the efficacy on the prevention of the immune response.

Drug Allergy in Type II Hypersensitivity

Type II hypersensitivity is a common cause of drug allergy. Hemolysis can occur when anti-drug antibodies, which are formed as described in type I hypersensitivity, recognize drug molecules, e.g., phenacetin and chlorpromazine, bound to the surface of erythrocytes. Such an antibody–hapten interaction will trigger either CMC or ADCC. Besides erythrocytes, platelets and granulocytes in the blood may also be affected by the antibody–drug interaction on the cell surface and cause thrombocytopenia and granulocytopenia, respectively. Another drug-related type II hypersensitivity is drug-induced autoimmunity. For example, drugs such as hydralazine, procainamide and isoniazid are capable of inducing antinuclear antibodies. The formation of antinuclear antibodies can develop lupus erythematosus syndrome. Another example of drug-induced autoimmunity is the administration of methyldopa. In a small portion of the population, the binding of methyldopa on the surface of erythrocytes will induce the formation of antibodies against erythrocyte surface antigens and result in an autoimmune response against erythrocytes. Generally, drug-induced type II hypersensitivity diminishes shortly after administration of the specific drug is discontinued.

Type III Hypersensitivity

Type III hypersensitivity, also known as immune complex hypersensitivity, is caused by the formation of antibody–antigen complexes in the blood or tissues. Although both type I and II hypersensitivities are also mediated via antibody–antigen interactions, there are cells involved in the initial stages of the reactions, i.e., IgE-associated mast cells and antigen-coated target cells, respectively. In type III hypersensitivity, the initial stage is the formation of soluble antibody–antigen complexes which are too small to be cleared by the reticuloendothelial system. These complexes will adhere to the surface of blood vessels or kidney glomerular tubes and subsequently cause tissue injury (Figure 5.5).

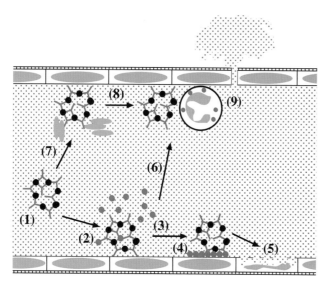

Figure 5.5. Type III or immune complex hypersensitivity. Immune complexes in the blood (1) will attach to the endothelium of the blood vessel (2), most likely in kidney glomerular tubes. The endothelial cell-associated immune complexes can bind C1 complement factors (2), activate the complement cascade reaction (3), promote the formation of membrane-attack complexes (4), and finally cause cell lysis (5). Endothelial cell-associated immune complexes can also attract platelets (7) and neutrophils (8). These cells can release vasodilators and cause leakage of endothelium (9).

The allergic response following the attachment of the immune complexes to the cell surface is similar to that of type II hypersensitivity; both complements and effector cells can be responsible for tissue injury and the release of anaphylatoxins and chemotactic factors that can cause inflammation. Type III hypersensitivity is especially detrimental to the kidney because immune complexes are easily trapped in the renal glomeruli which will cause glomerulonephritis. The condition of immune complex-associated symptoms is known as serum sickness.

Immune complexes can form locally when antigens contact the body at sites other than in the blood. In fact, the intradermal injection of antigens to test for the presence of antibodies, a test known as the Arthur reaction, is based on a local immune complex formation. In a postive Arthur reaction, a dermal inflammatory response appears 2 to 5 hours after the injection. Edema, erythema and hemorrhage are caused by the interaction of immune complexes with complement and, subsequently, neutrophils and monocytes infiltrate to the injection location. Inhaled antigens can cause type III hypersensitivity in the lungs. This type of allergic problem occurs in many occupational diseases as a result of pneumoconiosis. The common antigens are fungi in mold and animal proteins found in feathers, furs,

and feces. Workers who regularly inhale airborne antigens such as moldy dust in agricultural processes or tissue debris in animal handling may develop hypersensitivity within the alveoli in the lungs, a condition known as immune complex pneumonitis.

Drug Allergy in Type III Hypersensitivity

Serum sickness used to be a common side effect when antisera were used as the drug of choice for the treatment of infectious diseases and poisonous snake bites. Because of the development of antibiotics and active immunization, the administration of this type of treatment has become less frequent than before. Recently, hybridoma and recombinant DNA technologies have introduced monoclonal antibodies and cytokines as therapeutic agents for the treatment of various types of human diseases which could also invoke an immune response. Most of these recombinant protein drugs can only be administered by i.v. injection; therefore, their induction of hypersensitivity must be considered in clinical applications. Besides proteins, several small molecular drugs such as penicillin and procarbazine can also cause serum sickness-like reactions.

Type IV Hypersensitivity

Type IV hypersensitivity, also known as delayed-type hypersensitivity (DTH), is different from the other three types of hypersensitivity in that it does not involve antibodies in the reaction and takes more than 12 hours to develop allergic symptoms. The center of this immune reaction is interleukins that are secreted from T cells and macrophages in response to antigen challenge (Figure 5.1). When antigens first interact with T-lymphocytes, they initiate T cell activation and proliferation. These activated T cells, together with antigen-presenting cells, will secrete interleukins, particularly the macrophage activating factor, which will activate macrophages to kill microorganisms. Activated macrophages, however, may differentiate into giant cells and develop into granulomatous hypersensitivity, a form of DTH characterized by the formation of granulomas surrounded by insoluble suture materials. Many diseases such as tuberculosis and leprosy are associated with the development of granulomatous hypersensitivity.

Type IV hypersensitivity is also responsible for contact allergy such as common allergic reactions to poison ivy, cosmetics, clothing, etc. The antigens usually are highly reactive, small molecules which are capable of forming conjugates with constituents of the skin. Individuals who have previously been exposed to the antigen and have sensitized T cells will undergo an allergic response toward the same antigen in subsequent contact. This skin reaction begins approximately 24 hours after exposure and reaches

Type of drugs	Examples
Antibiotics and anti-infectious drugs	Penicillin, Sulfonamides, isoniazid
Antihypertensive drugs	Hydralazine, methyldopa
Antiarrhythmic drugs	Quinidine, procainamide
Antipsychotic drugs	Tricyclics, phenothiazines
Proteins and peptides	Hormones (e.g., insulin), enzymes (e.g., L-asparaginase)
Antibodies	Antisera, purified animal immunoglobulins or fragments, monoclonal antibodies

Table 5.5. Examples of drugs with potential allergic reactions.

a maximum between 2 to 4 days and is characterized by redness, induration and vesiculation.

Management of Drug Allergy

It is estimated that allergic reactions account for approximately 10% of all observed adverse drug side effects, and that 5% of all adults in the US may be allergic to one or more drugs (Table 5.5). In fact drug allergy is one of the major reasons for the exclusion of effective drugs in the treatment of human diseases (Table 5.6). Unfortunately, except for macromolecular drugs such as proteins and polysaccharides, it is difficult to identify an immunologic

Location of Reaction	Symptoms
Dermatological reaction	Erythema, edema
Respiratory reaction	Asthma
Hematological reaction	Hemolytic anemia, eosinophilia, immune cytopenia
Hepatic reaction	Cholestasis
Renal reaction	Glomerulonephritis
Systemic reaction	Anaphylaxis, serum sickness, lupus erythematosus

Table 5.6. Common symptoms of drug allergic reactions.

Before the prescription of a drug:

Avoiding overprescription of unnecessary drugs

Avoiding, if possible, drugs that are known to cause allergic reaction.

Assessing the drug history of the patient, especially on structually related drugs.

Before the administration of a drug:

Performing the skin test if possible.

Designing a dose schedule.

After the occurrence of drug allergy:

Informing the patient if a drug allergic reaction is identified.

Keeping medical records on drug allergic reactions.

Informing FDA of any newly identified drug allergic reactions.

Table 5.7. Prevention of drug allergy.

mechanism that is responsible for the reaction toward a specific drug that causes an allergy. It is generally believed that a small molecular drug or its metabolite cannot induce immune responses unless it can bind covalently to a protein carrier. Drug-macromolecular conjugates can be immunogenic and can elicit the formation of anti-hapten antibodies against the structure of the drug. There are also drugs that can either cause the degranulation in mast cells (type I hypersensitivity) or induce the autoimmune response to erythrocytes (type II hypersensitivity); therefore, the occurrence of drug allergic reactions as related to immunological mechanisms is still unpredictable at the present time, making the prevention of drug allergy a largely unsolved problem. Nevertheless, though, there are several guidelines that have been suggested by allergists for avoiding clinical problems related to drug allergy (Table 5.7).

Generally, drugs that are known to cause allergic reactions should be avoided if possible. In the case where there is no alternative drug for the treatment, the allergic reaction may be predetermined by assessing the drug history of the patient, such as previous administration of the specific or a structurally related drug. Furthermore, an allergy screening test such as the skin test for penicillin can be performed. Patients should be informed if a drug allergic reaction to a drug is identified so that the future exposure to the same drug can be avoided. Information regarding the patient's drug allergy should also be described in all of his or her medical records.

There are several principles that can be applied to minimize the incidence of a drug allergy. The administration route can be critical in inducing allergic reactions. Generally, the oral route is least likely to elicit an allergic response to an antigen, and smaller doses are also less likely to cause allergic reactions; therefore, a small dose can be given initially with increments over a period of time in order to determine the safe dose for a specific drug. Finally, if an allergy causing drug must be administered to a patient, an immune suppressor can be co-administered. This method is used when protein drugs are administered repeatedly to patients, such as the injection of anti-T lymphocyte antibodies for the prevention of graft-rejection in organ transplantation. ■

References

- **Baldo BA, Pham NH.** (1994). Structure-activity studies on drug-induced anaphylactic reactions. *Chem Res Toxicol*, **7**, 703–721
- **Bochner BS, Undem BJ, Lichtenstein LM.** (1994). Immunological Aspects of Allergic Asthma. *Ann Rev Immunol*, **12**, 295–335
- **Busse WW.** (1994). Role of antihistamines in allergic disease. *Ann Allergy*, **72**, 371–375
- **Canadian Society of Allergy and Clinical Immunology.** (1995). Guidelines for the use of allergen immunotherapy. *Can Med Assoc J*, **152**, 1413–1419
- **De Vries JE.** (1994). Novel fundamental approaches to intervening in IgE-mediated allergic diseases. *J Invest Dermatol*, **102**, 141–144
- **Fireman P, Slavin RG, eds.** (1991). *Atlas of Allergies*. New York, New York: Lippincott
- **Korenblat PE, Wedner HJ.** (1992). *Allergy — Theory and Practice*, 2nd ed. Philadelphia, PA: W.B. Saunders Co.
- **Lichtenstein LM.** (1993). Allergy and the immune system. *Sci Am*, **269**, 117–124
- **Lichtenstein LM, Fauci AS.** (1992). *Curr Ther Allergy, Immunol, and Rheumatol*, 4th ed. New York, New York: B.C. Decker
- **Rieder MJ.** (1993). Immunopharmacology and adverse drug reactions. *J Clin Pharmacol*, **33**, 316–323
- **Van Arsdel PP Jr.** (1991). Drug Allergy. *Immunol Allergy Clin N Am*, **11(3)**, 461–700

Case Study with Self-Assessment Questions

DM is a 37 year old industrial engineer, who was is his usual state of health prior to admission. After eating his dinner, he began to develop abdominal cramps and pains that radiated to the right flank and epigastric area. He was taken to the hospital and was diagnosed to have possible rupture appendicitis with possible peritonitis and bacteremia. Upon admission, DM was taken into surgery for appendectomy.

His post-operative course was complicated with cellulitis at the incisional site two days after the surgery. DMs medical history was positive for penicillin allergies which precluded the used of penicillins and first generation cephalosporins. Alternative therapy was to give the patient vancomycin at 1 g every 12 hours, as an intravenous injection.

The vancomycin was admixed in 250 ml of Dextrose 5%, and the infusion rate was 10 ml/minute (600 ml/hr). Within 10 minutes of infusion, the patient developed an intense erythematous rash that spread from his neck to his face and scalp. The rash then progressed to his upper chest and upper extremities. Accompanying the rash was intense pruritus. Hemodynamically, the patients blood pressure dropped to 98/57, as compared to a baseline measurement of 122/78. Other vital signs were as follows: Heart rate 110, respiratory rate 29, and core temperature of 38.4°C.

Question 1: *What clinical measures should be enacted to manage the patients drug reactions?*

Question 2: *Is vancomycin a wrong choice of antibiotic for a patient who is allergic to penicillin?*

Question 3: *From the described signs and symptoms, what type of hypersensitivity reaction is this patient most likely experiencing?*

Answer 1: Rapid infusion of vancomycin can cause the release of histamine from eosinophils. Thus reducing the rate of infusion from 10 ml/minute (600 ml/hr) to 4 ml/min (250 ml/hr) may reduce the risk of developing cutaneous reaction. However, it is possible that the patient is allergic to vancomycin due to previously unknown hypersensitization to this or other structurally related drug. In the latter case, reducing infusion rate may not alleviate the symptoms; the administration of vancomycin should be stopped and an alternative antibiotic should be used.

Answer 2: This is a correct choice for a patient who is allergic to penicillin because vancomycin is structurally different from beta lactams.

Answer 3: As described in (1), vancomycin can cause the release of histamine from eosinophils. Therefore, the patient may experience a pseudo-allergic reaction which is not mediated by immunological reactions. However, if the patient is indeed allergic to vancomycin, both type I and II hypersensitivity can produce similar symptoms, and require similar treatment.

6 Humoral and Cellular Immunodeficiency

Introduction to Immunodeficiency

Inability to respond adequately to an antigen intrusion is usually considered an immunodeficiency, whereby the immune system is unable to neutralize or eliminate the pathogen. Immunodeficiency occurs when one or more immune compartments are significantly affected, and are characterized by partial or complete impairment. When immune function is partially impaired, the term immune dysfunction is often used. Immune function disorders can be classified as humoral (B-cell mediated), cellular (T-cell mediated), combined immunodeficiency, phagocytic dysfunction disorders or complement deficiencies.

The emergence of acquired immunodeficiency syndrome (AIDS) has highlighted the importance of a completely intact immune system. Various causes or "triggers" of immunodeficiency include chemical, autoimmune, malignancy, and viral mediated syndromes. These disparate causes accentuate the paradigm that the various components of the immune system must work in concert to orchestrate a defense against foreign invasion.

Humoral immunodeficiency includes individuals who produce either an inadequate quantity of antibodies or non-functional antibodies. Pre-term infants and patients with chronic lymphoblastic leukemia (CLL) are examples of individuals who may have low concentrations of antibodies, or hypogammaglobulinemia. These individuals are susceptible to pyrogenic or bacterial infections. Alternatively, patients with cellular immunodeficiency such as patients with cyclic neutropenia, severe combined immunodeficiency (SCID), and HIV are susceptible to opportunistic infections such as *Pneumocystis carinii* and *cryptococcus neoformans*. Advances in our understanding of the immune system have increased survival in patients who no longer succumb quickly to their primary disease. Immuno-deficiency disorders are listed in Table 6.1.

Immune Disorder	Molecular basis of immunodeficiency	Clinical manifestation
X-Linked Agammaglobulinemia (X-LA)	Inability to form mature plasma cells	Low IgG, recurrent bacterial infections
Selective IgA Deficiency	Defect in HLA-A1, HLA-B8, and HLA-D expression	Recurrent infections, gastrointestinal disorders, autoimmune syndromes, allergic reaction, and malignancies development
Common variable immunodeficiency (CVID)	Defect in ability to synthesize and/or secretion of immunoglobulin	Autoimmune defect, increase autoantibodies, and hypogammaglobulinemia
DiGeorge syndrome	Abnormal embryonic development of 3rd and 4th pharyngeal pouches	Unable to produce mature and functional T-lymphocytes
Wiskott-Aldrich syndrome (WAS)	Defective cellular surface CD43	Reduced T- and B-cells, low Ig, anergic response, and recurrent infections
Severe combined immunodeficiency disease (SCID)	Genetic defect on chromosomal Xq11-13	Susceptible opportunistic infections
Adenosine deaminase deficiency (ADA deficiency)	A point mutation or deletion of the ADA gene	Susceptible to infections and autoimmune disease

Table 6.1. Immunodeficiency disorders.

Humoral Immune Dysfunction

In general, individuals who have reduced levels of either antibodies and complement are associated with increased risk of bacterial infections. The reduction of these humoral factors will impair the ability to opsonize pathogens such as *Streptococcus pneumoniae* or *Hemophilus influenzae*. Low levels of immunoglobulin may account for the inability to neutralize antigens and recruit a cellular response. However, patients with multiple myeloma, who have high levels of antibodies, are also susceptible to recurrent pneumococcal infections. Here the importance of antigen specific antibodies or functional antibodies is well illustrated. Therefore, both antibody concentrations and specificity are crucial in the process of eliminating pathogenic invasion.

X-Linked Agammaglobulinemia

B-cells are derived from stem cells that mature into lymphoid progenitor cells. These lymphoid progenitor cells can form either T- or B-lymphocytes. The factors which influence the formation of either T- or B-cells have still to be determined. However cytokines such as interleukins and interferons seem to play an important role in regulating normal cellular differentiation, maturation, and activation of lymphocytes.

X-linked agammaglobulinemia (X-LA) is an autosomal recessive genetic disorder found primarily in males. This B-cell immunodeficiency is characterized by low levels of IgG due to a defect in normal lymphocyte development or lymphopoiesis. Pre-B-lymphocytes derived from X-LA patients are unable to differentiate into mature B-lymphocytes or plasma cells, which are important in antibody production. There are two possible causes of this disorder, where affected patients are unable to form lymphoid progenitor cells and/or produce inadequate cytokine signals that are required for differentiation.

Patients with X-LA are usually diagnosed between 5 and 36 months of age. Clinically, these patients develop recurrent bacterial sinusitis or pulmonary infections caused by *Streptococcus sp, Staphylococcus sp, Escherichia coli*, and *Hemophilus influenzae*. Although these infections are common in this age range, X-LA patients are also susceptible to viral and protozoal infections despite having adequate numbers of circulating T-cells with normal function.

Selective IgA Deficiency

IgA is an immunoglobulin that is found primarily in secretions such as saliva, tears, mucosa, bronchial, vaginal, and prostatic fluids. Areas where IgA is found include the mucosa of the gastrointestinal tract. As described in Chapter 2, the primary role of IgA is to provide local defense against foreign substances before the antigen can enter into the body or circulation.

IgA deficiency (IgA-D) is the most common primary immunodeficiency. Unlike other humoral disorders, patients with IgA deficiency may not have any clinical manifestation of the condition due to adequate immune compensation where IgG and IgM concentrations are increased. Clinical manifestations may include recurrent infections, gastrointestinal disorders, autoimmune syndromes, allergic diseases, and malignancies. Patients with IgA-D may have serum IgA levels that are below 5 mg/dL.

Although the etiology of this immunodeficiency is still unclear, there is evidence suggesting a defect in human leukocyte antigen (HLA) expression. Defects of HLA-A1, HLA-B8, and HLA-D expression have been linked to the clinical manifestation. These include decreased numbers of circulating B-lymphocytes that are able to synthesize IgA. In addition, these lymphocytes are unable to secrete immunoglobulins across the epithelium into the extracellular space. Thus, primary IgA-D may be an immunodeficiency caused by the inability to secrete immunoglobulin to the affected site.

Common Variable Immunodeficiency

Common variable immunodeficiency (CVID) is a primary B-lymphocyte deficiency syndrome that is characterized by low levels of serum immunoglobulin, where levels of IgG are <250 mg/dL. Levels may be low in one or more classes of immunoglobulin. However, low levels of immunoglobulin cannot be explained by reduced numbers of circulating B-cells. Patients with CVID can have low, normal or above normal levels of circulating B-cells. This would suggest that the etiology of this disorder may be attributed to either defective immunoglobulin synthesis or secretion.

Other causes of CVID have been attributed to increased numbers of suppressor T-cells, which may suppress B-lymphocyte maturation into plasma cells. When patients are initially diagnosed with CVID, the number of circulating T-cells may be normal. However, there is a progressive decline of regulatory T-cells (Helper T-lymphocyte) with disease progression. These findings led to the hypothesis that CVID may be mediated by viral infections such as Epstein-Barr virus (EBV). Clinical presentation of these patients supports the viral-mediated etiology in that these patients may develop an autoimmune defect, followed by high levels of circulating autoantibodies, and viral-associated hypogammaglobulinemia.

Cellular Immunodeficiency Syndromes

In contrast to humoral immunodeficiency who are generally more susceptible to bacterial infections, patients with T-cell immunodeficiencies are susceptible to viral and fungal infections. They are at risk for severe reactions to childhood disease such as chickenpox (Varicella zoster) and measles. These individuals are also at risk of developing acute infections following vaccination with live attenuated vaccines, because of their inadequate immune capacity to prevent the subacute infection from regaining its original virulence. In addition, individuals with cellular immunodeficiencies are more likely to develop graft versus host disease-like (GvHD-like) reactions after transfusion(s) contaminated with lymphocytes or allogeneic hematopoietic stem cells.

DiGeorge Syndrome

DiGeorge syndrome is a T-lymphocyte immunodeficiency caused by abnormal development of the third and fourth pharyngeal pouches during embryogenesis. Between the sixth and tenth week of gestation, the thymus, parathyroid, thyroid, heart and certain facial features are developed. Thus, environmental or chemical insult during this period can lead to abnormal development of pharyngeal pouches. The complete or partial absence of the thymus can lead to the formation of defective T-lymphocytes.

The thymus is vital in T-lymphocyte maturation, where immature T-cells migrate from the bone marrow to the thymus. When lymphocytes have entered into the thymic environment, various stimulatory signals and cytokines will influence the development of immature precurors into mature T-lymphocytes. Thus, patients with DiGeorge syndrome are unable to produce mature and functional T-lymphocytes. This is evident by the lack of T-cell receptors (TCR or CD3) on the surface of circulating lymphocytes in patients with DiGeorge syndrome, suggesting that even the most primitive T-cells are not developed. Antibody levels are often normal in these patients; however, the majority of these antibodies are non-specific where T-cell dependent antibodies such as specific IgG are significantly depressed.

When patients with DiGeorge syndrome were treated with IL-2, immune function was restored. Before therapy, peripheral blood lymphocytes (PBLs) from these patients have undetectable levels of TCR subunits, α/β complex. However, TCR was normally expressed after 3 months of IL-2 therapy, which may explain the pathogenesis of DiGeorge syndrome. Moreover, the administration of IL-2 seems to mimic the thymic environment that promotes T-cell maturation.

Wiskott-Aldrich Syndrome

Wiskott-Aldrich syndrome (WAS) is an autosomal recessive disorder that is seen primarily in males who develop thrombocytopenia, eczema, and recurrent pyogenic infections. WAS is caused by the inability to produce antibodies directed against polysaccharide antigens. The pathogenesis

of this syndrome is thought to be caused by a defect in a cell surface glycoprotein known as CD43, sialophorin, leukosalin, or sialoglycoprotein. This surface cell marker is a sialic acid rich glycoprotein. However, the role of CD43 in WAS is still unclear. Macrophages and platelets in patients with WAS have abnormal granules which prevent normal antigen processing for presentation to T-cells. Inability to process antigen will inhibit T-cell activation, thus leading to both B- and T-lymphocyte immunodeficiency.

At birth, WAS patients have normal lymphocyte counts, but a decline in circulating lymphocytes is seen with advancing age. More specifically, lymphocyte decline is accompanied by a drop in the number of helper T-cells along with an abnormal CD4/CD8 ratio. Furthermore, these lymphocytes do not respond to antigenic stimuli. Later stages of WAS can clinically present as markedly reduced T- and B-cells, low serum immunoglobulin, anergic response to exposed antigens, and recurrent infections.

Severe Combined Immunodeficiency Disease

Severe combined immunodeficiency disease (SCID) is another autosomal disorder, which has been genetically mapped to chromosome Xq11-13. Patients with SCID have profound immunodeficiency of both T- and B-cell lineages. Severe lymphopenia is a hallmark of SCID, where lymphocytes bearing CD3, CD4, and CD8 are significantly diminished or absent. In addition, B-cells are also absent, with little to no antibody response to immunization. Individuals with SCID are also susceptible to opportunistic infections such as *Pneumocystis carinii* pneumonia (PCP). Moreover, patients with SCID may develop GvHD due to maternal transfer of immunocompetent lymphocytes through the placenta. Another possible method of induction of GvHD is blood transfusions contaminated with lymphocytes. This can be prevented by irradiating all blood products to prevent the transfer of lymphocytes into the infants with SCID.

The only treatment for SCID is allogeneic transplantation in the hope that the immune system can be reconstituted using donor bone marrow. The identification of the specific genetic defect has also enabled the development of methods to deliver the correct, wild type gene(s) into stem cells. Such gene therapy may provide the means for a cure of this deadly disease.

Adenosine Deaminase Deficiency

Adenosine deaminase (ADA) is an enzyme that catalyzes the conversion of adenosine and 2'-deoxyadenosine (dAdo) to inosine and 2'-deoxyinosine in normal purine metabolism. The absence of ADA activity will cause an accumulation of dAdo in body fluids and tissue. When dAdo is phosphorylated to deoxy-ATP, this can act as an inhibitor of DNA synthesis, resulting in cell death. The principal site where ADA deficiency is manifested is in T-lymphocytes; however, B-cells are also affected. The molecular mechanism of ADA deficiency has been traced to either a point mutation or deletion of the ADA gene.

The identification of a genetic mutation in patients with ADA deficiency has provided important insights into strategies to treat this disorder. One such therapy includes bone marrow transplantation where allogeneic stem cells have a functional ADA gene. Unfortunately, allogeneic BMT has significant morbidity associated with this type of treatment. Thus, another therapeutic modality must be developed. Irradiated red blood cell (RBC) transfusions, a rich supply of ADA, have been used to treat patients with ADA. Other alternatives have included bovine ADA conjugated with polyethylene glycol (PEG-ADA) which proved to be effective in reducing levels of dAdo. PEG-ADA provides several advantages over irradiated RBCs in that it eliminates the adverse effects related to transfusion. In addition, PEG conjugation prolongs ADA elimination thus decreasing the frequency of administration.

Future therapeutic modalities will include the insertion of a wild type ADA gene into the patient's own stem cells. The expression of normal ADA is expected to provide a cure in these patients. However, methods to deliver and maintain gene expression continue to challenge researchers.

Phagocytic Dysfunction

Circulating phagocytes consist of cells derived primarily from neutrophilic and monocytic lineages. Impaired ability to phagocytose foreign agents can emanate from either extrinsic or intrinsic factors. Hypogammaglobulinemia or complement deficiency are examples of extrinsic factors, where levels of these humoral factors are inadequate to activate phagocytic chemotaxis and localization to the affected site. Other extrinsic factors include decreased levels of chemoattractants or cytokines such as interleukin-8 (IL-8). Intrinsic phagocytic dysfunction can be caused by a defect in metabolic pathways such as myeloperoxidase production. Absence or deficiency in myeloperoxidase will cause a delayed antibacterial and antifungal activity.

Complement Dysfunction

Complements are important humoral factors for opsonization of antigens and initiating chemotaxis. Deficiencies in complement factors can lead to recurrent pyrogenic infections and increased risk for autoimmune disorders. Glomerulonephritis and systemic lupus erythematosus (SLE) have been associated with low levels of complement components, such as C1, C4, and C2.

C3 and C5 are important in immune adherence, opsonization, chemotaxis, and activating the inflammatory response. The absence of C3 increases the risk of developing bacterial infections, similar to patients with hypogammaglobulinemia, whereas functional deficiency of C5 leads to intractable diarrhea, recurrent fungal and gram-negative bacterial infections. A deficiency in C5, C6, and C7 can lead patients to develop disseminated *Neisseria gonorrhoeae* or meningitis.

Virus-Mediated Acquired Immunodeficiency Syndrome

In the early 1980s, Kaposi's sarcoma (a vascular tumor that occurs predominately in elderly men) and *Pneumocystis carinii* pneumonia (PCP) were found in homosexual men who had severe immunodeficiency. The causative agent was later found to be a retrovirus that was initially called human T-lymphotropic virus-III (HTLV-III) or lymphadenopathy virus (LAV). This virus was later renamed human immunodeficiency virus (HIV).

Human immunodeficiency virus (HIV) is a retrovirus that utilizes ribonucleic acid (RNA) as its genetic blueprint for cellular replication and protein synthesis, instead of deoxyribonucleic acid (DNA). Biologically, HIV is like a cellular parasite where the infected cell serves as a host. Following infection, the RNA template is converted into DNA code or complement DNA (cDNA) (Figure 6.1). This

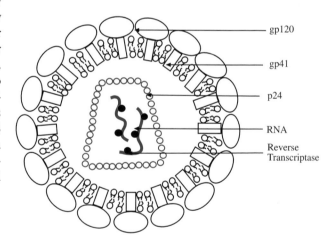

Figure 6.1. The structure of the HIV is composed of a major surface agent that is primary glycoprotein 120 kDal or gp120. gp120 is anchored onto the cellular membrane by a glycoprotein that is 41 kDal, also known as gp41. HIV has an intercore protein covering all the nucleocapside which is made up of a protein that has a molecular weight of 24 kDal (p24). Within the nucleocapside is the genomic RNA and reverse transcriptase that translate the RNA into a DNA code.

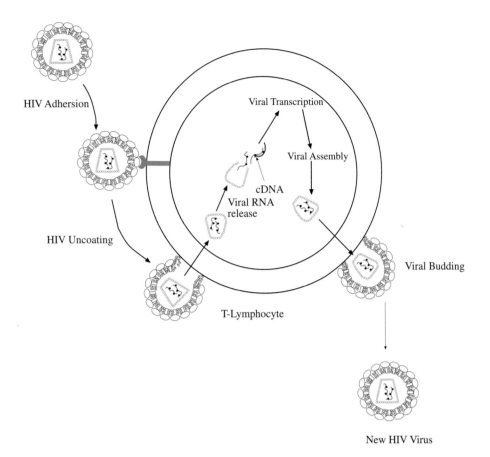

Figure 6.2. After gaining entry into the host, the HIV surface antigen, gp120, binds onto the CD4 receptor of the host cell. The binding onto the CD4 cell allows the membranes of HIV and host cells to exchange phospholipids, and thus gain entry into the host. The viral RNA is released into the cytoplasm of the host cells, where complement DNA is formed. Once the viral DNA is formed, transcription of viral proteins may take place to form the new virons.

is accomplished with the aid of reverse transcriptase (RT), which is unique to retroviruses, and thus has become a target to inhibit HIV.

There are four major HIV genomes that are referred to as *gag* (structural proteins), *pol* (polymerase), *env* (envelope glycoproteins), and *tat* (transactivatory of transcription). The *tat* and *gag* genes have been shown to be important in the facilitating the transcription of viral genome and viral assembly, respectively, and have been the target for many antiviral agents.

How Does the HIV Infect CD4+ Cells?

The major surface antigen on HIV is gp 120 (glycoprotein 120 kDa). This glycoprotein is anchored onto a transmembrane glycoprotein also referred to as gp41 (Figure 6.2). Inside HIV is a protein capsule or nucleocapside that protects the viral genome. The nucleocapsule is composed of a 24 kD protein also known as p24. Inside this nuclear protein capsule is the genetic material composed of RNA and RT.

After the virus has gained access to the circulation, the HIV adheres to the CD4 complex using gp120, and enters the host cell by fusing onto the CD4 cell membrane. Once the membranes have merged, the viral RNA is converted to complement DNA (cDNA). An anti-complement strand of DNA is then formed to give rise to double-stranded DNA. The double-stranded DNA can either circularize or be incorporated into the host's genetic material by means of HIV integrase. Once viral DNA is corporated into the host cell, viral activation occurs following cytokine activation (such as IL-1, IL-3, IL-6, TNF, and GM-CSF). The elevation of pro-inflammatory mediators occurs following antigen induction, or through a response against HIV progression.

When HIV is activated and viral transcription occurs, viral precursor protein such as *gag-pol* protein is formed. Gag-pol protein is an inactive precursor protein that requires proteolytic cleavage to form the active proteins, such as viral proteases, p24, reverse transcriptase, and integrase. Once active proteins are formed, assembly into infectious particles can take place.

Clinically, HIV infected patients may not progress to full-blown AIDS for as long as 7–10 years. Progression of HIV infection to AIDS is thought to be prevented by lymph node sequestration. The virus is sequestered in the germinal centers of the lymph nodes, where cellular immunity mediated by NK and CTLs will control viral dissemination into the circulation. Viral destruction can lead to accumulation of cellular debris within the lymph nodes, where blockage of the lymph nodes may clinically present as enlargement of lymph nodes or lymphadenopathy. Following viral breakdown of lymph node sequestration, the HIV will enter into the circulation, thus permitting the virus to infect circulating CD4 cells. Progression to AIDS occurs when the HIV has caused a decline in CD4 cells to less than 200 cell/mm³, indicating the presence of significant immunodeficiency. A patient can also be classified as having AIDS when the HIV infected patient is found to be infected with opportunistic infections or present AIDS-related malignancies. These AIDS defining illness include *Pneumocystis carinii*, *Toxoplasma gondii*, *Cryptococcus neoformans*, viral herpes, AIDS-related lymphomas, and Kaposi's sarcoma.

Early progression to AIDS carries a poor prognosis for long-term survival, where patients may have a life expectancy of months rather than of years. Most HIV infected patients can remain asymptomatic for years until their CD4 cell counts drop below 200 cell/mm³. As HIV proliferation progresses, there is a continual deterioration of the immune system. This is evident from bone marrow suppression or pancytopenia. Most notable of this myelosuppressive activity is lymphopenia or, more specifically, a decline in helper T-lymphocytes (CD4-lymphocytes). Although a drop in CD4-bearing cells is observed, a reduction in CD8 cells is also noted. CD4-lymphocyte reduction may be attributed to two factors: 1) direct viral lysis and 2) cytokine down-regulation by the secretion of IL-10, a T-cell inhibitory cytokine. In addition, viral infection can induce a high level of IL-4 expression that can turn off the expression of IL-2, IFN-γ and IL-12 that upregulates cellular immunity. As the level of IL-10 increases, an inverse relationship in IL-2 levels and CD4 cells is observed. As IL-4 and IL-10 increase, cellular immunity is suppressed thus allowing HIV to proliferate freely.

Immune Response to HIV Infection

There are three primary phases in HIV infection. The first clinical sign of HIV infection may include a acute flu-like syndrome followed by an asymptomatic phase. The third and final stage of HIV infection is the progression to full-blown AIDS, where the infected individual either develops opportunistic infections, AIDS-related malignancies, or immunodeficiency as evidenced by CD4 counts fall below 200 cells/mm³.

One of the biggest mysteries surrounding HIV infection is the conversion from asymptomatic HIV infection to full-blown AIDS. Factors inducing disease progression are not well delineated. These may include viral virulence and immune capacity to control viral proliferation. Another possibility includes co-factors or co-infections which may induce disease progression.

There are several hypotheses regarding AIDS progression. These revolve around the ability of HIV to induce an immune response. One hypothesis suggests that HIV infection can downregulate cellular immunity by reducing the number of T_{H1}-CD4 cells. The downregulation of T_{H1} is accompanied by an enhanced humoral response controlled by T_{H2}-CD4 cells (Figure 6.3), referred to as "immune switching." More importantly, T_{H2}-CD4 cells are susceptible to HIV proliferation.

HIV patients who have been infected for a long period and have not converted to full blown AIDS have normal numbers of T-cells and no dysfunction in cytotoxic activity. T-cells derived from these patients are able to produce and express high levels of IL-2 in response to HIV. In addition, such patients have minimal antibody production directed against HIV. However, in HIV infected patients with high levels of anti-HIV antibodies, only 50% of individuals are able to produce normal levels of IL-2. Cell-mediated activities are more effective in controlling HIV, than in patients with an elevated humoral response. Thus, a high level of IL-2 is able to maintain a T_{H1}-type response, which may be immunoprotective against progression to full-blown AIDS.

In individuals where IL-2 production is decreased, there is an inverse correlation with increased production and expression of IL-4, a modulator of T_{H2}-CD4. As expected, an increased production of IL-4 coincides with increased T_{H2}-CD4 with accompanying decrease in T_{H1}-CD4. The switching from T_{H1} to T_{H2} also correlates well with clinical progression to AIDS. Furthermore, an elevation of T_{H2} corresponds with an increase of IL-4 and IL-10 production, which can inhibit cellular immune activation.

One explanation why patients with T_{H1} mediated responses do not convert to full blown AIDS is that T_{H1}-CD4 cells are resistant to HIV infection, whereas T_{H2} are susceptible to HIV, allowing them to proliferate. Therefore HIV infection can create an environment where the immune system cannot stop its progression, and the immune cells that are mobilized are susceptible to HIV infection. Along with T_H cell switching, patients with HIV produce high levels of cytokines, such as GM-CSF and IL-6, which are able to activate HIV *tat* gene, and thus enhance viral proliferation.

During clinical progression to AIDS, patients lose their antigenic response to which they have been previously exposed. This is also known as anergy. This is caused by a loss of memory CD4 T-lymphocytes that can induce a more rapid immune response to previous antigenic expo-

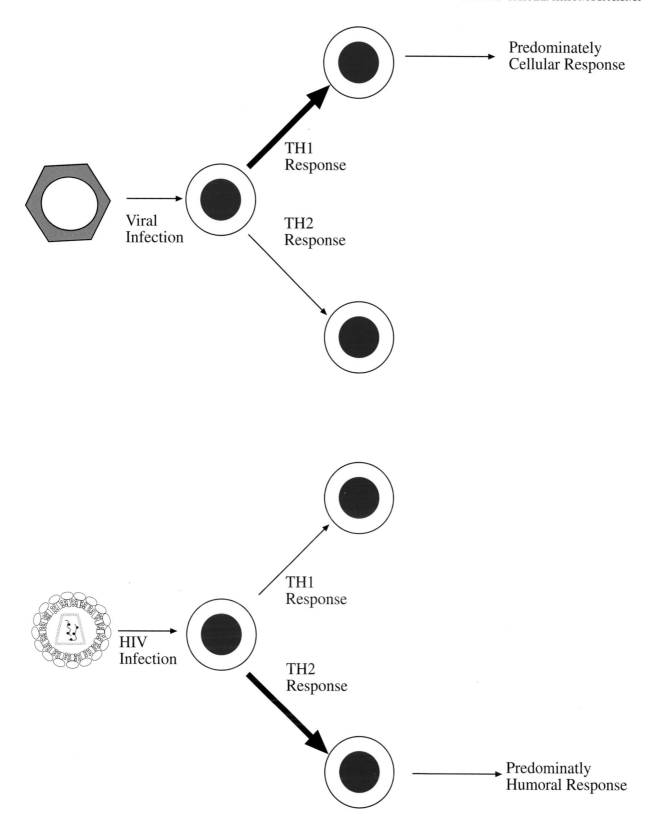

Figure 6.3. HIV-induced T_{H1} to T_{H2} immune cell switching. In event of a viral infection, T_{H1} is the primary response where expansion of CTLs is initiated. However, in HIV infection, there is a downregulation of T_{H1}. This is accompanied by an elevation of T_{H2}-CD4 cells which control humoral immunity, and susceptible to HIV infection.

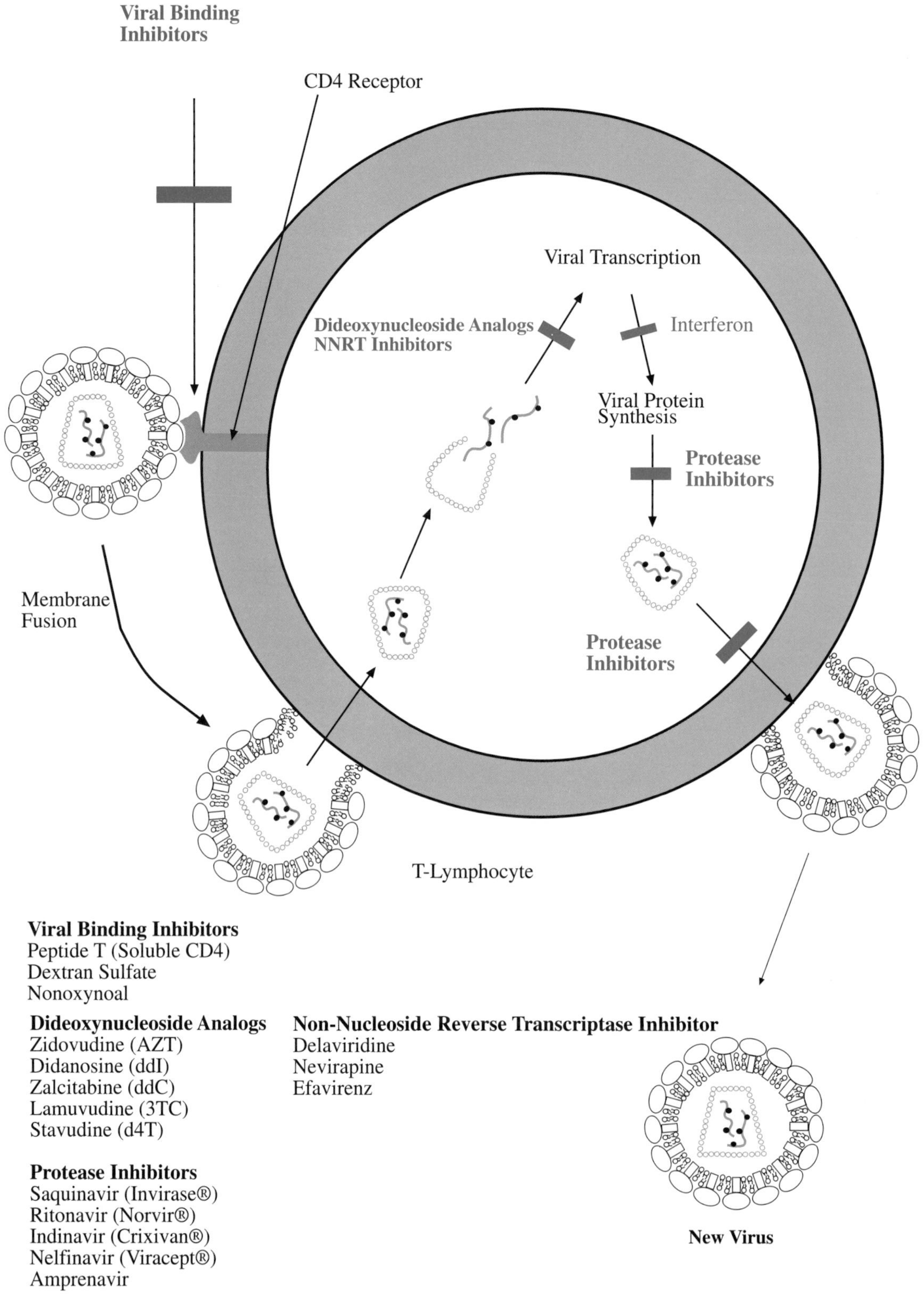

Viral Binding Inhibitors

CD4 Receptor

Viral Transcription

Dideoxynucleoside Analogs NNRT Inhibitors

Interferon

Viral Protein Synthesis

Protease Inhibitors

Protease Inhibitors

Membrane Fusion

T-Lymphocyte

Viral Binding Inhibitors
Peptide T (Soluble CD4)
Dextran Sulfate
Nonoxynoal

Dideoxynucleoside Analogs
Zidovudine (AZT)
Didanosine (ddI)
Zalcitabine (ddC)
Lamuvudine (3TC)
Stavudine (d4T)

Non-Nucleoside Reverse Transcriptase Inhibitor
Delaviridine
Nevirapine
Efavirenz

Protease Inhibitors
Saquinavir (Invirase®)
Ritonavir (Norvir®)
Indinavir (Crixivan®)
Nelfinavir (Viracept®)
Amprenavir

New Virus

Figure 6.4. There are various strategies to inhibit viral replication. 1) The inhibition of HIV binding onto the CD4 receptor prevents initial viral infection. 2) Both dideoxynucleoside analogs and non-nucleoside (NNRT) inhibitors prevent the formation of complement DNA. Protease inhibitors block the formation of active viral proteins by competitively inhibiting viral proteolytic enzymes.

sure. On the cellular level, a notable increase in naïve T-cells (T_{Ho}-CD4 cells) with a decline in T_{H2}-CD4 cells has been observed. T_{Ho}-CD4 are T-lymphocytes that are uncommitted to either T_{H1} or T_{H2}, and are able to produce and secrete cytokines produced by these helper T-cell subtypes. The conversion from T_{H1} to T_{Ho} may explain the loss of antigen recall. The depletion of T_{H2} may be due to viral lysis of infected cells. However, these two explanations do not totally explain the shift to T_{Ho}.

Clinical Sequelae of HIV Progression

The decline of CD4 cells is important because it correlates with clinical presentation. More recently, the decline in CD4 cells has been correlated with an increased HIV load, which initiates the decline of CD4 cells. As CD4 cell numbers drop below 500 cells/mm³, the incidence of Kaposi's sarcoma and AIDS-related lymphoma (non-Hodgkin's lymphoma) increases dramatically. When the CD4 count drops below 200 cell/mm³, the risk of developing opportunistic infections increases substantially. Infections such as *Pneumocystis carinii* pneumonia, *Toxoplasma gondii*, *Cryptococcus neoformans*, *Candida* sp, Cytomegalovirus, *Cryptosporium* sp, *Microsporium* sp. Cytomegalovirus, Herpes simplex and *Varicella-zoster* may also reactivate in patients who have been previous exposed. In HIV infected females, clinical manifestation may include recurrent vaginitis or development of venereal warts. All these are signs and symptoms of immune breakdown, where the host defense is unable to control pathogens that are in the environment from developing into clinical disease.

Clinical Treatment for HIV

Strategies for the prevention and treatment of HIV infection have concentrated on intervention at various stages in the HIV life-cycle. These include blocking the viral binding onto the CD4 receptor, inhibition of reverse transcriptase

(RT), inhibition of mRNA translation of viral protein, and inhibition of viral assembly and budding (Figure 6.4). Only by avoiding high risk activities or the development of an effective vaccination will the incidence of HIV infection decline. Prevention of HIV acquisition includes the use of condoms and engagement in safe-sex activities. These efforts have significantly reduced the incidence of new reports of HIV infection in the United States. The development of an effective vaccine is still a high priority in the fight to reduce HIV infection. This is especially important for individuals who are at risk for HIV exposure, such as healthcare workers, intravenous drug users, and individuals who engage in promiscuous or high risk sexual activity.

Genomic mapping studies have shown a high level of HIV variability. This frequently occurs in the *env* genome that encodes for cell surface glycoproteins, gp120 and gp41. Both conserved and variable regions within this genome exist; CD4 binding regions are highly conserved. In contrast, hypervariable regions thought to be mutational regions are utilized by HIV to evade the immune system. The identification of conserved regions within the gp120 structure has been a primary focus for vaccine development against HIV.

ANTIVIRAL THERAPY

Attempts to eradicate or inhibit the progression of human immunodeficiency virus (HIV) have focused primarily on interfering with the HIV replication cycle. Therapeutic agents include those that block HIV binding onto CD4 cells, reverse transcriptase inhibitors, and protease inhibitors.

The majority of commercially available antiviral agents have targeted viral reverse transcriptase (RT) and protease inhibitors. Currently, the treatment to prevent HIV progression is the use of dideoxynucleoside analogs, such as zidovudine (AZT), didanosine (ddI), zalcitabine (ddC), stavudine (d4T) and lamivudine (3TC). The pharmacological profiles of these agents are summarized in Table 6.2. The mechanism of action of dideoxynucleoside analogs is

Agent	Dose	F	Tmax	T1/2	Prot Bind	Vdss
Zidovudine (AZT)	100 mg PO 5X/day 200 mg PO TID	0.63	0.6–0.8 h	1 h	34–38%	1.3–1.6 l/kg.
Didanosine (DDI)	200 mg PO BID >60 kg 125 mg PO BID <60 kg	0.3	0.6–1 h	1.3–1.6 h	<5%	45l.
Zalcitabine (DDC)	0.75 mg PO BID	0.8	0.8 h	1–3 h		0.5–0.6 l/hr.
Lamivudine (3TC)	150 mg BID PO	0.82	1 h	2.5 h	<36%	1.3 l/kg.
Stavudine (D4T)	0.5 mg/kg/day. 40 mg BID PO	0.8	0.5–1.5 h	1–1.6 h		

Table 6.2. Pharmacokinetics of dideoxynucleoside analogs.

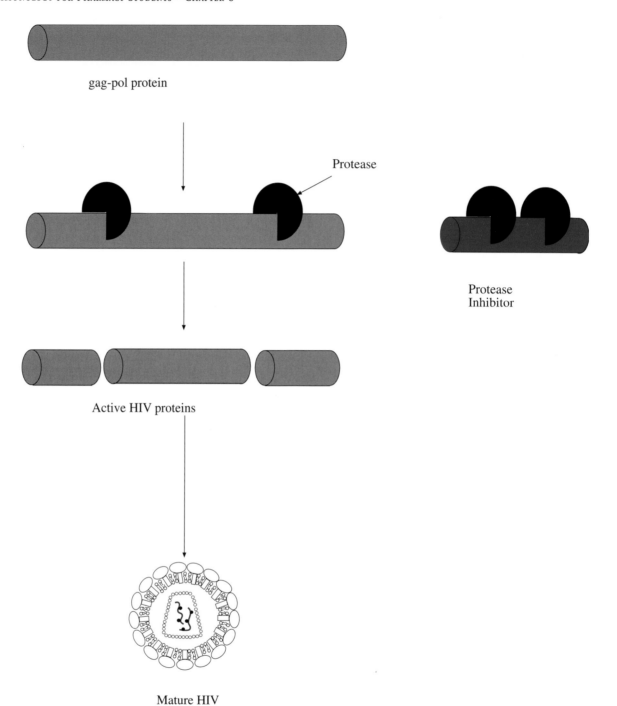

gag-pol protein

Protease

Protease
Inhibitor

Active HIV proteins

Mature HIV

Figure 6.5. HIV protease inhibitors exert their antiviral activity through blockade of viral protease enzymes in a competitive reversible fashion. HIV proteases are inhibited. These are essential to form active building blocks for the developing infectious HIV particles.

to inhibit viral DNA (cDNA) elongation; these agents lack the 3'-hydroxyl group on the ribose moiety that is required for DNA elongation (Figure 6.4). Although, initial studies have shown that reverse transcriptase inhibitors were able

to prolong survival, recent data disputes findings as to the efficacy the dideoxynucleoside analog.

These agents are not without adverse effects. AZT is associated with neutropenia. In contrast, patients taking

	Saquinavir	Indinavir	Ritonavir	Nelfinavir
Bioavailability	4% (12–16% SG)	14–70%	70–90%	70–90%
Half-life	1.5 hour		3–4 hour	3.5–5 hour
Vd	700 L	3x body water		
Protein binding	98%	15–56%	99%	≤98%
Dosage	600 mg TID	800 mg TID	600 mg BID	750 mg TID
VIC	12 µg/L	50 nM	2.1 µg/mL	800 µM
Plasma conc (Average)	35 µg/L		5–10 µg/mL	3–4 µg/mL

Table 6.3. Pharmacokinetic profiles of FDA approved protease inhibitors.

ddC, ddI, d4T, and 3TC rarely develop hematological disorders. Rather, individuals receiving these agents usually exhibit peripheral neuropathy and pancreatitis as their major adverse effects (Table 6.5). Other adverse effects include nausea, vomiting, and diarrhea.

The regulatory agencies have approved the use of another class of drugs called HIV protease inhibitors. Protease inhibitors should be used in combination with dideoxynucleoside analogs. Monotherapy using protease inhibitors alone is discouraged, because of the rapid development of resistance. These agents work primarily through blockade of viral protease enzymes, in a reversible fashion. HIV proteases are essential for the formation of active protein building blocks to form mature and infectious HIV particles (Figure 6.5).

During the biosynthetic stages of HIV, viral proteins such as *gag-pol* polypeptides are formed. Gag-pol protein precursor has no biological activity in its native form. Active viral building blocks are formed when HIV proteases enzymatic cleave the gag-pol protein to its active form. The gag-pol protein precursor contains the amino acid sequence of various HIV protein components such as capsid (p19) and nucleocapsid (p24). In addition, gag-pol protein also contains the amino sequence for all retroviral enzymes, such as reverse transcriptase, proteases, and integrase. Integrase facilitates viral genome integration into the host DNA, thus allowing the virus to take over host cellular machinery.

Protease inhibitors are agents that resemble pieces of protein that competitively binds onto HIV enzyme or protease. This reversible binding reduces the number of enzymes that are involved in formation of active HIV proteins.

Currently there are four protease inhibitors that have received regulatory agencies' approval (Table 6.3). These agents are approved for use in combination with dideoxy-

Most frequently reported adverse events	Frequency of adverse effect
Diarrhea	3.8%
Abdominal discomfort	1.3%
Nausea	1.9%
Abdominal pain	1.9%
Buccal mucosa ulceration	2.5%
Asthenia	1.3%
Rash	1.3%

Table 6.4. Adverse efects associated with protease inhibitors.

nucleoside analogs. A number of other protease inhibitors are also on the verge of gaining approval.

Unlike other protease inhibitors, nelfinavir has a favourable bioavailability profile. The bioavailability of protease inhibitors has been a concern for the drugs that have already received commercial approval. These results are summarized in Table 6.3.

Despite the lack of definitive information, protease inhibitors have been approved due their ability to reduce HIV viral load. Significant antiviral and clinical effects have been achieved using protease inhibitors when combined with dideoxynucleoside analogs.

Ritonavir is the first protease inhibitor to show that patients receiving triple antiviral combination can improve their survival time and delay opportunistic infections. This was demonstrated in 1090 volunteers with advanced HIV disease (CD4 $\geq$ 100). At the beginning of the study, the median HIV plasma viral load was over 250,000 viral/mL. After six months, a 43% reduction in mortality was seen in patients receiving ritonavir as compared to placebo (patients received 2 dideoxynucleoside analogs). Ritonavir therapy for six months was able to reduce the incidence of opportunistic infections and death by 64%. This may be attributed to a reduced viral load, which can decline to 96% of baseline levels in patients receiving protease inhibitors. Viral reduction was however not maintained and returned to baseline despite continued therapy.

Indinavir is similar to ritonavir in terms of antiviral activity, but is better tolerated due to its reduced gastrointestinal side effects. Unlike ritonavir, indinavir should be taken on an empty stomach to maximize absorption. The combination of indinavir with two nucleoside analogs (AZT + 3TC) were able to suppress viral load below undetectable for longer than 100 weeks.

Saquinavir *in vitro* has the best anti-HIV activity. However, only 4% of the oral dose is absorbed and this has limited its utility. Recent studies have employed the use of a newer oral formulation which has an improved bioavailability where the bioavailability is 12–16%. An alternative means of increasing saquinavir level is to one way to increase bioavailability is to combine saquinavir with ritonavir which is able to increase blood levels of saquinavir.

SIDE EFFECTS AND DRUG INTERACTIONS OF PROTEASE INHIBITORS

No direct comparisons have been made between the four potent protease inhibitors. The antiviral activity reported for these drugs may appear to be very similar, but their side effects and drug interactions are different (Table 6.4 & 6.5).

Ritonavir appears to be the least well tolerated. In one study, which used the traditional liquid formulation, three-quarters of the study participants experienced nausea. More than half developed diarrhea, and more than a quarter had episodes of vomiting, causing one-third of patients to eventually drop out of the study. Likewise, 17% of those receiving ritonavir at the clinical endpoint for advanced patients stopped taking the drug because of nausea, vomiting, weakness and diarrhea.

Fewer patients dropped out of the study when indinavir was employed, due to differences in the side effects profile. Patients taking indinavir developed elevated levels of bilirubin, but did not appear to have symptoms or discomfort. The dose limiting adverse effect of indinavir is nephrolithiasis which can be extremely painful. Some new side effects were reported in combination studies using indinavir with AZT/ddI, where indinavir therapy resulted in more cases of dry skin, insomnia, rash, pharyngitis and flank pain.

Nelfinavir caused grade I/II diarrhea, defined as two to six bowel movements per day in 70 to 100 percent of patients. Initially diarrhea was mild with patients' complaints being primarily of "soft stools."

Convenience of dosing is a factor to be taken into consideration when deciding on compliance issues. Ritonavir is advantageous in this respect, with twice-a-day dosing; however six capsules must be taken each time. Nelfinavir and saquinavir is dosed three times a day and can be taken with a little food. However indinavir has to be taken three times a day on an empty stomach, something which is difficult for patients with problems in keeping their weight stable.

One consideration when using protease inhibitors is that they have a powerful inhibitory effect on hepatic metabolism. Therefore when protease inhibitors are taken with medications requiring metabolism for their elimination, there is an increased risk of drug accumulation. Changes in drug metabolism can lead to drug interactions. Difficulties with protease inhibitors are encountered, where antibiotics used for prophylaxis and/or treatment cannot be used due to potential toxic drug interactions. The number of drugs that interact with the protease inhibits includes antimycobacterial, antiepileptic, antihypertensive, and long-acting non-sedative antihistamine agents.

Immune Therapy

Interleukin-12. Following HIV infection, evidence suggests that the virus can induce immune switching from a cell-mediated response (T_{H1}) to a humoral (T_{H2}) mediated response. Cytokine studies show that IL-4, IL-6 and IL-10 are all elevated in patients with HIV infection. In contrast, cytokines that stimulate T_{H1} were significantly decreased. These studies raise the question as to exogenous administration of T_{H1} cytokines, such as IL-2, IFN-γ, or IL-12, increasing cellular immunity to HIV progression. A stable T_{H1} response may induce a strong CTL response to HIV, while reducing the number of T_{H2} cells that may serve as an HIV reservoir.

The use of exogenous of IL-12 may reverse HIV-induced suppression of endogenous IL-12 production. IL-12 is predominantly produced by macrophages in response to pathogens, where the release of IL-12 stimulates CTL expansion and enhances cytolytic activity of NK cells. Furthermore, IL-12 can induce T-lymphocytes to increase production of IFN-γ, which is also a potent stimulator of the cellular response. *In vitro*, IL-12 can restore cell-mediated immunity against HIV, and cause a reduction of viral RNA. Not only is IL-12 a promoter of the T_{H1} cellular response, but it also inhibits IL-4 producing cells. That is, IL-12 may be effective in inducing a T_{H1} immune response, and thus may be more effective in combating HIV infection.

Drugs	Dose	Adverse Effects
Dideoxynucleoside analogs		
Zidovudine(AZT)	200 mg PO TID	Anemia, neutropenia, neuropathy, headaches, nausea, vomiting
Didanosine (DDI)	125 mg PO BID <60kg, 200 mg PO BID >60kg	Neuropathy, pancreatitis, and myelosuppression
Zalcitabine (DDC)	0.75 mg PO BID	Peripheral neuropathy, pancreatitis
Stavudine (D4T)	40 mg bid PO	Neuropathy, pancreatitis
Lamivudine (3TC)	150 mg bid PO	Rash, diarrhea and neuropathy
Protease inhibitors		
Indinavir (Crixivan)	800 mg po q8h	Nausea/vomiting/diarrhea, abdominal pain, headache, fatigue, kidney stones
Ritonavir (Norvir)	600 mg po bid	Nausea/vomiting/diarrhea, abdominal pain, Peripheral paresthesia, fatigue, taste disturbance anorexia
Saquinavir (Invirase)	600 mg po tid	Diarrhea, abdominal discomfort, nausea/vomiting/diarrhea
Nelfinavir (Viracept)	750 mg po tid	Diarrhea, headache, fatigue

Table 6.5. Treatment for HIV.

When any drug is being considered as a possible agent for human therapy, the toxicity associated with the treatment must be tolerable. IL-12 has similar toxicity profile as that of IL-2; low grade fevers, chills, malaise, myalgias and arthralgias are frequently encountered. However, the effectiveness in reducing viral load has not been conclusively been determined.

Interleukin-2. IL-2 has been used in tumor immunomodulation. In the early 1980s, IL-2 was given to patients with HIV to boost their immune system. Patients who were given IL-2 had high CD4 cell counts. Instead of an improved immune response against the HIV, these patients developed progressive AIDS and succumbed to their disease at 6 months after the initiation of IL-2 therapy. IL-2 increased the number of CD4 cells which are a reservoir for HIV infection. In addition, IL-2 is a potent stimulator of the *tat*-gene which can activate HIV proliferation. These two properties prevented the use of IL-2 alone to boost the immune system.

Recently, the use of IL-2 in HIV has been resurrected when it was combined with dideoxynucleoside analogs. The addition of dideoxynucleoside analogs along with IL-2 potentiates the antiviral effect of AZT, d4T, ddI, ddC, and 3TC. This was accomplished through IL-2-mediated enhancement of cellular phosphorylation of dideoxy-

nucleoside analogs to the active triphosphate agent. High levels of the triphosphate form of dideoxynucleosides increase viral DNA incorporation, resulting in termination of viral DNA synthesis.

Granulocyte Macrophage Colony Stimulating Factor. The combination of antiviral agents with cytokines such as GM-CSF has also been tested. Like IL-2, when GM-CSF is used alone, there is an increase in viral replication. However, when GM-CSF is given concomitantly with an antiviral such as AZT, an increased level of AZT-triphosphate (TP-AZT) is produced. There is a dose-dependent antiviral activity with intracellular levels of TP-AZT correlating with HIV inhibition. Although AZT and its metabolite, d4T, act synergistically with GM-CSF, there is antagonism when the dideoxynucleoside analogs ddI and ddC are used to prevent viral replication. The types of HIV therapy is summarized in Table 6.5.

Opportunistic Infections Associated with AIDS

TREATMENT OF HERPES VIRUS

As mentioned earlier, a decline in CD4 cells increases the risk of developing opportunistic infections. HIV patients who have been previously exposed to herpes infection may have a reactivation of their viral infection as the immune system deteriorates. Herpes virus is able to reactivate and proliferate when the immune system is no longer able to suppress viral disease. Patients with herpes reactivation will develop herpetic lesions similar to *de novo* infections. The lesions track along nerve dermatones wherein the virus resides.

Similarly, *de novo* herpetic infections usually clinically manifest with dermatological lesions along nerves. However, in immunodeficient patients who develop *de novo* infections may show involvement of visceral organs or viremia. The difference in clinical course may be attributed to the role of the immune system in preventing the progression of disease.

The primary treatment for herpes simplex is acyclovir which requires phosphorylation to the active triphosphate form. This requires thymidine kinase which is found at substantiately higher levels in herpes virus than in mammalian cells; thus viral infected cells more effectively transform acyclovir to acyclovir-triphosphate. The dose of acyclovir in the treatment of herpes simplex is 5 mg/kg every 8 hours by intravenous injection. Acyclovir can also be used in patients with reactivation of herpes varicella zoster or "chickenpox". However, the dose of acyclovir must be increased to 10 mg/kg every 8 hours.

Herpes infections are now easily treated with acyclovir. However, the use of acyclovir has also resulted in the emergence of acyclovir resistant herpes, also known as herpes simplex type VI (HSV-VI). When acyclovir resistant herpes is suspected, an alternative drug such as foscarnet is used. With foscarnet, a course of induction therapy must precede the maintenance therapy. Induction therapy is intravenous foscarnet given at 60 mg/kg every 8 hours for 14 days. The dose is then reduced during the maintenance phase, to 90–120 mg/kg given daily. Long-term use of foscarnet can cause electrolyte imbalance, and serum levels of Na, K, Ca, and Mg may be altered.

CYTOMEGALOVIRUS

Unlike other immunodeficiency patients, AIDS patients develop cytomegalovirus (CMV), primarily ocular. Patients with CMV usually have signs and symptoms that include fever, chills, weakness, and blurred vision. CMV retinitis can be identified by ophthalmological examination, revealing patchy lesions in the retina.

Laboratory tests may reveal an increase in the level of antibodies (or titers) directed against CMV. Patients with CMV retinitis can be effectively treated with ganciclovir (DHPG). Other alternatives include foscarnet at the same dosage that was used for the treatment of Type VI herpes infections. In patients with disseminated disease, it may be necessary to use combination therapy. The mortality rate

associated with disseminated CMV pneumonitis approaches 75% despite therapy using single-agent pharmacology. Combination of either ganciclovir or forcarnet with intravenous immunoglobulin has reduced mortality to 25%.

PNEUMOCYSTIS CARINII PNEUMONIA

The first groups of patients with HIV initially presented with a rare parasitic lung infection. *Pneumocystis carinii* pneumonia (PCP) clinically manifests as a dry cough, where some patients complain of a metallic taste. Their laboratory values may be notable for elevated lactate dehydrogenase (LDH), decreased oxygenation in arterial blood gase (ABG) tests and elevated Pco_2. A chest X-ray (CXR) is notable for patchy lung infiltrates. However, definitive diagnosis is made when sputum containing Pneumocystis is seen on microscopic examination. However the absence of PCP in the sputum does not exclude the parasite in the pathogenesis of the disease.

The treatment of PCP centers around the combination of trimethoprim/sulfamethoxazole (Bactrim and Septra). At doses of 15–20 mg/kg/day of the TMP component, these patients may experience significant adverse effects, including nausea, vomiting, neutropenia, kidney and liver dysfunction. Cutaneous reactions such as rash and itching are the most frequently encountered adverse effects. These cutaneous reactions have been attributed to allergies associated with sulfur containing drugs. There is evidence that cutaneous reactions are attributed to accumulation of sulfamethoxazole metabolites. Some patients may not be able to tolerate TMP/SMX (e.g. development of bone marrow suppression) and drug resistance is apparent. Alternative therapy may be necessary. The first alternative is to use intravenous pentamidine at 3–4 mg/kg/day intravenously. Pentamidine can also be administered via inhalation. Inhaled pentamidine can reduce systemic toxicity, which can be severe. Other alternatives include clindamycin and primaquine in combination, dapsone and TMP in combination and atovaquone. The prevention of PCP is one way to avoid the disease. Patients are given one double strength dose of trimethoprim/sulfamethoxazole. Inhaled pentamidine (300 mg monthly) can also be used to prevent PCP.

TOXOPLASMA GONDII

AIDS patients may also develop other parasitic infections such as *Toxoplasma gondii*. Clinical manifestation includes persistent headaches. Radiological tests such as computerized axial tomography (CAT) of the brain may reveal encapsulated lesion(s) which is a hallmark of Toxoplasma infection. The primary treatment for toxoplasmosis usually employs combination therapy consisting of pyrimethamine and sulfadiazine. Folinic acid is added to prevent sulfadiazine-induced hematological suppression. Alternative therapy may employ clindamycin containing regimens that may be used alone or in combination with other anti-toxoplasmosis agents. Clindamycin can be used in combination with pyrimethamine, thus allowing a dose of clindamycin of 300–600 mg every 8 hours. Clarithromycin and azithromycin are macrolide analogs of erythromycin with significant activity in toxoplasmosis.

CRYPTOCOCCUS NEOFORMANS

Central nervous system infections can present as headaches with accompanying chills and fevers. In patients with these symptoms, it is necessary to consider *Cryptococcus neoformans*. Patients with CNS cryptococcal infections must be initially treated with amphotericin B at 0.4–1.0 mg/kg/day. When amphotericin resistant strains of *Cryptococcus sp* are encountered, the addition of flucytosine (5FC) as a synergistic agent is necessary. Flucytosine is an analog of 5-fluorouracil (5FU), a chemotherapeutic agent, and may cause myelosuppression. An alternative treatment is azole analogs like fluconazole, itraconazole, and ketoconazole. Both itraconazole and ketoconazole do not penetrate adequately into the CSF, and their use is precluded in meningeal infection. Another obstacle to the use of azoles is that they are only fungistatic, i.e. the drug only inhibits fungal proliferation. Chronic therapy is necessary here to prevent clinical relapse, where chronic suppressive fluconazole is primarily used.

YEAST INFECTIONS

Oral fungal infections are one of the most commonly encountered opportunistic infections. Although such infections are easily treatable in the immunocompetent individuals, they can progress into life-threatening disease in HIV patients if untreated. There are a number of therapeutic options that include clotrimazole, nystatin, ketoconazole, itraconazole, and fluconazole. Yeast infections of the oral cavity can easily progress to esophagitis and even fungemia, and more aggressive therapy may be needed. The treatent of HIV-related opportunistic infections is summarized in Table 6.6. ■

References

- **Brunda MJ.** (1994). Interleukin-12. *J Leuk Biol*, **55**, 280–288
- **Chehim, J, Starr SE, Frank I,** *et al.* (1994). Impaired interleukin 12 production in human immunodeficiency virus-infected patients. *J Exp Med*, **179**, 1361–1366
- **Clerici M, Giorgi JV, Chou, C,** *et al.* (1992). Cell-mediated immune response to human immunodeficiency virus (HIV) type 1 in seronegative homosexual men with recent exposure to HIV. *J Infect Dis*, **165**, 1012–1019
- **Clerici M, Lucey DR, Berzofsky JA, Pinto LA,** *et al.* (1993). Restoration of HIV specific cell-mediated immune responses by interleukin-12 *in vitro*. *Science*, **262**, 1721–1724
- **Clerici M, Shearer GA.** (1993). A TH1 to TH2 switch is a critical step in the etiology of HIV infection. *Immunol Today*, **14**, 107–110
- **Fischl MA, Richmann DD, Grieco MH,** *et al.* (1987). The efficacy of azido-thymidine (AZT) in the treatment of patients with AIDS and AIDS-related complex: a double blind, placebo-controlled trial. *N Engl J Med*, **317**, 185–191
- **Hall SS.** (1994). IL-12 holds promise against cancer, glimmer of AIDS hope. *Science*, **263**, 1685–1686
- **Maggi E, Mazzetti M, Ravina A,** *et al.* (1994). Ability of HIV to promote a TH1 to TH0 shift and to replicate preferentially in TH2 and TH0 cells. *Science*, **265**, 244–251
- **Manetti R, Parronchi P, Giudizi MG,** *et al.* (1993). Natural killer cell stimulatory factor (Interleukin 12[IL-12]) induces T helper type 1 (TH1)-specific immune responses and inhibits the development of IL-4-producing TH cells. *J Exp Med*, **177**, 1199–1204
- **Mosmann TR.** (1994). Cytokine patterns during the progression to AIDS. *Science*, **265**, 193–194
- **Salk J, Bretscher PA, Salk PL,** *et al.* (1993). A strategic for prophylactic vaccination against HIV. *Science*, **260**, 1270–1272
- **Sirianni MC, Ansotegui IJ, Aiuti F, Wigzell H.** (1994). Natural killer cell stimulatory factor (NKSF)/IL-12 and cytolytic activities of PBL/NK cells from human immunodeficiency virus type-1 infected patients. *Scand J Immunol*, **40**, 83–86

Treatment	Major Toxicities
Pneumocystis carinii	
Trimethoprim/Sulfamethoxazole 15–20 mg/kg/day (in 3–4 divided doses) IV or PO for 2–4 weeks	Nausea, vomiting, rash, neutropenia, Thrombocytopenia, hepatitis, azotemia
Pentamidine 3–4 mg/kg/day IV qd for 21 days	Neutropenia, thrombocytopenia, hepatitis, azotemia, hypoglycemia
Aerosolized Pentamidine 4–8 mg/kg qd for 21 days	Bronchospasm, cough, bad taste
Dapsone 100 mg qd + Trimethoprim 20 mg/kg/day PO	Methemoglobinemia for G6PD deficiency
Clindamycin 900 mg q6–8h + Primaquine 30 mg PO QD	Diarrhea, pseudomembranous colitis, Myelosuppression, increased LFTs, GI upset
Trimetrexate 45 mg/m² IV QD for 21 days + Folinic acid 20 mg/m² PO or IV QID for 21 days	Neutropenia, nausea, vomiting
Toxoplasma gondii	
Pyrimethamine 50 mg LD, then 25 mg PO QD + Sulfadiazine 2 gm LD then 1–1.5 gm PO QID + Folinic acid 10 mg PO QD	Thrombocytopenia, neutropenia
Clindamycin 1200–1600 mg Q6–8H IV	GI upset, hepatotoxicity, C. difficule
Clarithromycin 500–1000 mg PO BID	GI-upset, nausea, vomiting and diarrhea
Histoplasmosis	
Amphotericin-B 0.5–0.6 mg/kg IV QD	Renal toxicity, fever, chills
Itraconazole 200 mg PO BID	Nausea , hypokalemia, hepatitis
Coccidiomycosis	
Amphotericin-B 0.5 mg/kg IV QD	Renal toxicity, fever, chills
Fluconazlole 400–800 mg QD	Nausea, vomiting, diarrhea
Cytomegalovirus	
Ganciclovir 5–7.5 mg/kg/q12h IV for 14 days, then 2.5–5 mg/kg/day	Granulocytopenia, nausea, vomiting, fever, psychosis
Foscarnet 60 mg/kg/q8h IV for 14–21 days, then 90–120 mg/kg IV QD	Neutropenia, electrolyte imbalance, nephrotoxicity
Immunoglobulin 500–1000 mg/kg for 2–7 days IV	Hypersensitivity reactions
Herpes Simplex	
Acyclovir (800 mg PO q8h or 5 mg/kg IV q8)	Crystalluria, CNS confusion
Foscarnet 60 mg/kg q8h for 21 days	Neutropenia, electrolyte imbalance, nephrotoxicity
Herpes Varicella-Zoster	
Acyclovir 10–12 mg/kg/q8h IV for 7–14 days	Crystalluria, CNS confusion
Famiciclovir 500 mg TID PO for 7–14 days	
Cryptococcus Neoformans	
Amphotericin B 0.3–0.6 mg/kg/day IV + Flucytosine 25–37.5 mg/kg/d PO in 4 doses	Renal toxicity, fever, chills, marrow suppression, elevated LFT's
Fluconazole 200–400 mg PO QD	GI upset, abdominal pain, increased LFTs
Itraconazole 200 mg PO BID	Nausea, gastric pain, and hypokalemia

Table 6.6. Treatment of HIV related opportunistic infections.

Case Studies with Self-Assessment Questions

Case 1

AM is a 2 year old male who has a history of recurrent bacterial and viral infections. He was a full term baby but developed recurrent infections requiring frequent hospitalization. His work-up revealed a persistent low white blood cell count, low despite the presence of bacterial and viral infections. Explain why AM is unable to respond against microorganism invasion, if you are told that he had a rare genetic disorder called Adenosine deaminase (ADA) syndrome.

Question 1: *What is Adenosine deaminase syndrome, and what is the cause of this immunodeficiency?*

Question 2: *Which component of the immune system is defective? Be specific about the various components of the immune system.*

Question 3: *What clinical measures can you use to manage this type of immunodeficiency?*

Question 4: *What are some experimental therapies available for these patients, and how effective are they? Also explain the mechanism of action for these experimental therapies.*

Answer 1: Adenosine deaminase (ADA) is an enzyme that catalyzes the conversion of adenosine and 2'-deoxyadenosine (dAdo) to inosine and 2'-deoxyinosine in normal purine metabolism. The lack of ADA activity will cause an accumulation of dAdo in body fluids and tissue. dAdo is phosphorylated to deoxyATP which can act as an inhibitor of DNA synthesis, causing cell death. The principal site where ADA deficiency mediates its toxicity is in T-lymphocytes; however B-cells are also affected. The molecular mechanism of ADA deficiency was traced to either a point mutation or deletion of the ADA gene.

Answer 2: ADA deficiency causes a T-lymphocyte depletion, thus a lymphopenia is expected. A dysfunction in the lymphocytes can alter cytokine release that may affect other components of the immune system such as myeloid cells. Thus a depression in the white blood cell count is usually seen in patients with ADA deficiency.

Answer 3: The only FDA approved product is bovine ADA conjugated with polyethylene glycol (PEG-ADA) which has proved to be effective in reducing levels of dAdo. PEG-ADA provides several advantages over irradiated RBCs in that it eliminates the transfusion-related adverse effects. In addition, PEG conjugation prolongs ADA elimination, thus decreasing the frequency of administration.

Answer 4: Future therapeutic modalities will include the insertion of the ADA gene into the patient's own stem cells. The expression of normal ADA is expected to cure these patients.

Case 2

WY is a 26 year old female who was admitted for persistent chills, fevers, and dry cough. Her medical history was notable for numerous episodes of sexually transmitted diseases. Her last episode of STD was about 6 months ago, at which time she was treated with a course of ceftriaxone and doxycycline for gonorrhea and chlamydia, respectively. Other notable history included intravenous drug use with heroin and cocaine.

Her hospital admitting laboratory results were notable for low total white blood cell counts (WBC) and neutrophils. Chest X-ray revealed bilateral patchy infiltrates, consistent for *Pneumocystis carinii* pneumonia (PCP). Additional laboratory tests were ordered, which included CD4 counts and polymerase chain reaction (PCR) for human immunodeficiency virus (HIV). The HIV-PCR was positive for HIV, where WY had a CD4 counts of 24 cells/mL. A working diagnosis of HIV/AIDS was started and patient was started on trimethoprim/sulfamethoxazole for presumptive PCP.

Question 1: *What is the drug of choice for PCP? Would you change the pharmacological regimen if the patient were allergic to sulfur drugs?*

Question 2: *The patient is now stabilized with anti-Pneumocystis agents for her PCP. What type of anti-HIV retroviral therapy would be used? Explain your answer.*

Question 3: *If this patient develops cytomegalovirus, what is the drug of choice?*

Answer 1: Trimethroprim/sulfamethoxazole (TMP/SMX) is the drug of choice for patients with PCP. However, there are individuals who are allergic to sulfur agents like SMX. This precludes the use of TMP/SMX. In this case, pentamidine at 3–4 mg/kg given intravenously daily, would be an alternative agent for PCP.

Answer 2: Most recent studies suggest that patients with HIV and opportunistic infections should start on a triple combination consisting of zidovudine (AZT), lamuvudine (3TC), and a protease inhibitor (indinavir, ritonavir, or saquinavir). Triple antiviral therapy should be employed in patients whose CD4 cells are below 200 cells/mL.

Answer 3: Patients who develop cytomegaloviral infections should be placed on induction therapy. The drug of choice is ganciclovir at 5 mg/kg every 12 hours for 14 days. Following induction therapy, cytomegalovirus infections are suppressed by maintenance therapy using ganciclovir 5 mg/kg given daily. In patients who are intolerant to or develop resistance towards ganciclovir, foscarnet is recommended. Induction with foscarnet is 60 mg/kg every 8 hours for 14 days, followed by maintenance therapy at 90–120 mg/kg given once daily.

7 Cytokines and Immunotherapy

Introduction

The regulation of cells in the immune system is directly influenced by cytokines, also known as hematopoietic growth factors (HGF). Lymphokines, like interleukins (IL-1-14 except 3) and interferons (α, β, γ), regulate the activation, proliferation, and survival of lymphocytes. The biological activity of the lymphokines is shown in Table 7.1. Most notable of these interleukins is IL-2, which possesses antitumor activity by stimulating cytotoxic T-lymphocytes (CTLs) and natural killer (NK) cells. IL-4 has also been shown to increase CTL and NK activity, and is presently being tested in combination with IL-2. A B-cell growth factor like IL-6, that has myeloid cell regulatory activity.

Unlike other stimulatory cytokines, IL-10 is able to downregulate the immune system through inhibiting the expression of inflammatory cytokines such as IL-1 and tumor necrosis factor (TNF). With this biological activity profile, IL-10 is now being evaluated as a potential candidate for the treatment for autoimmune diseases. Some lymphokines may have myeloid cell regulatory activity such as IL-11 which is able to regulate platelets. IL-12 or natural killer cell factor is now being investigated as a possible agent to eradicate HIV infected cells. Thus the administration of exogenous cytokines can modulate or influence the biological activity of various tissues and cells, and is better known as "immunomodulation" or "immune therapy". In this chapter, an overview of how cytokines can alter the immune system will be highlighted.

Interleukins

Interleukin-2

Interleukin-2 (IL-2) is a lymphokine that has been shown to enhance cellular immunity, particularly cytotoxic T-lymphocytes (CTLs) and natural killer (NK) cell activity. IL-2 is a 133 amino acid glycoprotein with a MW of 15.4 kDa. When lymphocytes are stimulated with IL-2, they are referred to as lymphokine activated killer (LAK) cells because of their cytotoxic activity against both tumor lines and fresh autologous tumors. The institution of high doses of IL-2 (≥100, 000 units/kg every 8 hours) can stimulate the immune system to attack tumors in the body. The antitumor activity is attributed to the expansion of CTLs and NK cells. IL-2 can also mobilize both NK cells and CTLs, such that they can be harvested through a process called leukapheresis. In this process, the entire blood volume is systematically removed and centrifuged to separate the various components. When the spin direction of the centrifuge is changed, the separated cells can be harvested.

Stimulated lymphocytes and NK cells can be expanded and maintained in culture in the presence of IL-2. After stimulation with IL-2, the activated lymphocyte can be infused back into the patient. The transfusion of activated white cells is accompanied by administration of high doses of IL-2 to maintain the stimulated state. When high dose of IL-2 and LAK cells are used in combination, a 90% response is achieved in patients who have metastatic (disseminated) renal cell carcinoma. The favorable response rate using IL-2 and LAK in disseminated renal cell carcinoma is because these patients have already failed other conventional and salvage therapy. When this combination is tried in other tumors, the response rate is less dramatic. IL-2 and LAK only produce a 50% clinical response in patients with metastatic melanoma; the response rate (30%) for metastatic colon cancer is even poorer.

Due to the high cost of maintaining and expanding LAK cells in culture, the efficacy of LAK cells in combination with rhIL-2 was compared to high dose rhIL-2 alone. Initially, patients receiving both LAK cells and high dose IL-2 have better survival rates than IL-2 alone. However, long-term patient survival was not significantly different between the groups receiving IL-2 with LAK as compared to IL-2 alone. This study highlighted the fact that no advantage could be gained from adding LAK cells.

Despite eliminating LAK cells, the IL-2 dosage used in patients with renal cell carcinoma is associated with severe adverse effects. These side effects are related to IL-2-induced capillary leakage syndrome. This process is caused by lymphocytes gaining access to the tumor. In order for this to occur, lymphocytes must leave the circulation and infiltrate the affected site. Small holes are formed along the vasculature when the lymphocytes infiltrate into the tissues. However the holes created will also allow intravascular fluids to escape into the extracellular space, which

Lymphokines	Biological activity
Interleukin-1	Primary inflammatory mediator that activates cytokine release, activation of immune cascade.
Interleukin-2	Primary T-cell activator that increase the activity of cytotoxic T-lymphocytes and natural killer cells.
Interleukin-4	Activate the maturation of B-lymphocytes to antibody producing plasma cells. Able to increase MHC class II expression on resting B-cells.
Interleukin-5	Activate B-lymphocyte maturation and stimulate eosinophil differentiation.
Interleukin-6	B-lymphocyte growth factor that influence the maturation of B-cells into plasma cells. Increase expression of antibodies.
Interleukin-7	B-lymphocyte growth factor
Interleukin-8	Neutrophil and T-lymphocyte chemotactic factor, with angiogenic properties
Interleukin-9	Secreted by activated T-lymphocytes with pleuritropic activity on serveral hematopoietic cells.
Interleukin-10	T-cell inhibitory cytokine which is able to inhibit TH1 cytokines such as IL-2 IFN-γ and IL-12.
Interleukin-11	Megakaryocyte factor
Interleukin-12	Cytotoxic T-lymphocyte and natural killer cell factor that is able to enhance cytolytic activity.
Interleukin-13	Exact physiological role is still unclear
Interleukin-14	Exact physiological role is still unclear
Interleukin-15	T-lymphocyte factor
Interferon-α	T-lymphocyte factor in response to viral infection and foreign intrusion
Interferon-β	T-lymphocyte factor that increase expression of MHC class I expression on natural killer cells
Interferon-γ	Leukocyte factor produced in response to viral infection and the presence of tumors. Able to increase the expression of both MHC class I and II.

Table 7.1. Biological activity of lymphokines.

may explain why patients receiving IL-2 can develop peripheral edema and cardiopulmonary effusions. Intravascular fluid leaving the vasculature will reduce the volume required to maintain blood pressure, thus hypotension is also apparent in patients receiving IL-2 infusion (Table 7.2). In order to maintain blood pressure, it may be necessary to employ adrenergic agonists and vasopressors such as dopamine, dobutamine, and phenylephrine. Other IL-2 induced side effects include flu-like symptoms like chills and fevers that may be caused by rhIL-2-induced expression of TNF, interferon-gamma (IFN-γ), and IL-1.

IL-2 toxicities are dose related, thus efforts to reduce IL-2 have been explored. However, the antitumor activity of IL-2 is also dose-dependent. In an effort to reduce toxicity, lower doses of IL-2 have been employed in combination with IFN where the combination has been shown to be synergistic in the treatment of melanoma. Combination with other cytokines such as IL-4, a B-lymphocyte growth factor that is capable of enhancing CTL cytotoxic activity, has been shown to be effective in reducing IL-2-induced toxicities without reducing antitumor activity. IL-2 is also used in patients receiving tumor vaccines to

High doses of IL-2
• Hypotension
• Renal dysfunction
• Peripheral edema
• Epidermis exfoliation
• Retina detachment
• Pulmonary and pericardial effusion
Low doses of IL-2
• Chills
• fevers
• Malaise
• Myalgias
• Arthralgias

Table 7.2. IL-2 toxicities.

enhance immune recognition and response to the tumor antigen.

Interferons

As described in Chapter 1, interferons (IFNs) are cytokines that induce non-specific resistance to viral infections. They are classified into three major groups: alpha (α), beta (β), and gamma (γ). IFN-α is derived from leukocytes, whereas IFN-β and -IFN-γ is derived from fibroblasts and lymphocytes, respectively. IFNs exert their biological activity by inducing the expression of various viral inhibitory enzymes.

IFNs are produced when a cell is either sensitized by a pathogen or infected with a virus. Induction of IFN expression can be achieved artificially with double stranded RNA and poly (I:C), a polyinosinate and polycytodinate RNA chain. The presence of double stranded RNA may indicate the presence of a viral infection. Interferons were first identified in 1957, when cells exposed to inactivated viruses were able to produce a soluble factor that inhibited viral replication. The ability to "interfere" viral or "viron" replication gave rise to its name.

IFNs exert their antitumor activity primarily through activation of the cellular immunity and induction of target cell expression of MHC class I antigen. Cellular activity includes: 1) expansion of NK cells; 2) increased CTL activity; 3) enhanced macrophage phagocytic activity; and 4) increased antibody-dependent cell-mediated cytotoxicity. The induction of MHC class I antigen on the target cell will enable immune cells to recognize them as foreign cells, and mount an immunological attack on them.

There is some speculation that the antitumor activity of IFN may be a consequence of its viral inhibitory capabilities. Tumors that have been linked to viral infections include hepatocellular carcinoma (Hepatitis B, C and D), naso-pharyngeal carcinoma (Epstein-Barr virus), AIDS-related lymphomas, and AIDS-associated Kaposi's sarcoma (Herpes virus VIII). In addition, IFNs also have anti-proliferative and antiangiogenesis (inhibition of the formation of new blood vessels) which may add to its anti-tumor activity, especially in solid tumors.

Interferon-α

Human recombinant IFN-α (rhIFN-α) is commercially available for the treatment of hairy cell leukemia, condylomata accuminata, AIDS-related Kaposi's sarcoma, and chronic hepatitis. All of these disorders have been linked to viral infections (Table 7.3). Hairy cell leukemia is associated with human T-lymphotropic virus II (HTLV-II), whereas condylomata accuminata or venereal wart is associated with human papilloma virus. These viruses are oncogenic (capable of transforming infected cells into malignant growth).

The mechanism of action of IFN-α is thought to inhibit viral replication. Virally transformed cells can induce expression of mitogenic cytokines that can promote tumor proliferation. The inhibition of viral proliferation will directly inhibit the proliferation of transformed cells and the expression of tumor promoting growth factors. Furthermore, there is evidence that IFN-α is able to inhibit formation of new capillaries (antiangiogenesis). As the cancer grows, it will need new capillaries to supply the necessary nutrition. Ability to inhibit angiogenesis may explain why IFN-α is able to inhibit Kaposi's sarcoma, a highly vascularized malignant growth, seen primarily in males with HIV. IFN seem to be able to inhibit basic fibroblast growth factor and vascular endothelial growth factor, both which are important to promote angiogenesis. IFN-α is also able to inhibit mitogenic cytokines such as IL-6 and oncostatin M.

MULTIPLE MYELOMA

Multiple myeloma is a B-lymphocyte malignancy where in high levels of non-functional monoclonal antibodies are produced. Similar to Kaposi's sarcoma, multiple myeloma have been associated with herpes virus 8 (HSV-8), which may explain why IFN-α is effective against multiple myeloma,

Virus	Tumor
Hepatitis B	Hepatocellular carcinoma
Hepatitis C	Hepatocellular carcinoma
Human T-lymphotropic virus I	Acute T-cell lymphoma/leukemia
Human T-lymphotropic virus II	Hairy cell leukemia
Human immunodeficiency virus	AIDS-related lymphoma
Herpes virus VIII	AIDS-related Kaposi's sarcoma, Multiple myeloma
Epstein-Barr virus	Nasal pharygneal carcinoma, Burkitt's lymphoma
Human papilloma virus	Cervical, penile and rectal cancer

Table 7.3. Tumors that are linked to viral infections.

where expression of IL-6 is inhibited. The modulation of IL-6 production may be just one means whereby IFN exerts it antitumor activity. Other immunomodulatory activity may be activation of NK cells and CTLs. In addition, IFNs enhance tumor expression of MHC class I, thereby allowing NK cells and CTL's to recognize and eliminate tumor cells.

ACUTE T-CELL LEUKEMIA AND LYMPHOMA

Acute T-cell leukemia/lymphoma (ATL) and mycosis fungoides are diseases that are associated with human T-cell leukemia virus I (HTLV I) infections. Clinical presentation include 1) hypercalcemia, 2) elevated parathyroid hormone (PTH), 3) elevated CD4$^+$ cells, 4) CD4$^+$ cells acting like suppressor T-cell, and 5) elevated IL-10 levels. HTLV I is a retrovirus that can be transmitted through sexual contact, similar to HIV. When the infected cells are transformed, it leads to development of leukemia or lymphoma cells. ATL cells express high levels of IL-10, a T-cell inhibitory cytokine, that suppresses the expansion of CTLs and NK cells. This may explain why ATL patients are immunocompromised and susceptible to opportunistic infections. These immunological changes mimic the clinical presentation one would see in HIV, where patients with acute T-cell leukemia are susceptible to *Pneumocystis carinii* pneumonia (PCP).

At the present, there is no effective cytotoxic chemotherapeutic treatment for HTLV-I-linked ATL. However, there is substantial clinical response when moderately cytotoxic antiviral therapy is used in this disease. A combination of IFN-α with zidovudine (AZT) was able to produce complete remission (CR) with a sustained disease free survival of greater than 5 years. This is a significant discovery because ATL is usually refractory to any treatment,

including high dose chemotherapy and bone marrow transplantation. Other treatments are able to produce responses; however, these responses are not maintained and 5 year survival is less than 10%.

Interferon-β

The spectrum of activity of IFN-β is similar to that of IFN-α. This is understandable because both IFN-α and IFN-β bind to the same cell receptor. IFN-β 2b (Betasteron®) has obtained approved for the treatment of multiple sclerosis, an autoimmune disorder. Unlike IFN-α, IFN-β is able to downregulate T-cell activation. This is accomplished through downmodulation of IFN-γ, TNF-α, and lymphotoxin (TNF-β). In addition, patients receiving IFN-β are able to produce high levels of transforming growth factor β (TGF-β), a cytokine with immunosuppressive activity. Similar to IFN-α, IFN-β is active against a wide range of tumor lines including gliomas, breast cancer, and bladder cancer. Although IFN-β has anti-tumor activity, the full spectrum of activity is still unclear.

Interferon-γ

Recombinant human IFN-γ (Actimmune®) has been approved for the treatment of chronic granulomatous disease, an autoimmune disease that primarily affects the lungs. Although IFN-γ shares many functional properties that are found in IFN-α and -β, it differs in that it has better antiproliferative properties compared to other IFNs. This may be due to IFN-γ's ability to both stimulate expression of MHC class II on monocytes, and increase expression of MHC I on targeted cells. Similar to other IFNs, IFN-γ exerts its anti-autoimmune effect through reduction of

Interferon	Type	Company	FDA approved uses
IFN-α	IFN-α 2a (Roferon) IFN-α 2b (Intron) IFN-α N (Alferon) IFN-α Consensus	Roche Schering Amgen	Hairy cell leukemia, Hepatitis B and C virus, AIDS-related Kaposi's sarcoma, Chronic myelogenous leukemia, Condylomata acuminata, Multiple myeloma, Melanoma
IFN-β	IFN-β 2b	Chiron/Berlex Biogen	Multiple sclerosis
IFN-γ	IFN-γ (Actimmune)	Genentech	Chronic granulomatous disease

Table 7.4. Clinical uses for interferons.

Myeloid growth factors	CFU-GM	CFU-GEMM	CFU-E	BFU-E	CFU-Meg
M-CSF	+	−	−	−	−
G-CSF	+	−	−	−	−
EPO	−	−	+	+	−
TPO	−	−	−	−	+
GM-CSF	+	+	−	−	−
IL-3	+	+	−	−	+

Table 7.5. Activity of CSF.

pro-inflammatory mediators like TNF, IL-1 and IL-2. Clinical uses for interferons are given in Table 7.4.

Colony Stimulating Factors

Colony stimulation factors (CSFs) are hematopoietic growth factors (HGFs) that regulate the commitment, proliferation, maturation and function of myeloid cells. CSFs are primarily produced by either stimulated T-lymphocytes or macrophages. However, endothelial cells and fibroblasts have also been described as expressing CSFs during inflammatory events. Despite their overlapping biological activities, each CSF has its own distinctive structure; there is little structural homology between CSFs. Table 7.5 shows CSF activity, and adverse effects associated with CSFs are listed in Table 7.6.

Chemotherapy Induced Neutropenia

Cytotoxic antineoplastic agents used in the treatment of cancers are unable to discriminate tumor and self. Inability to selectively kill tumor cells can lead to a number of

Types of adverse effects	rhG-CSF	rhGM-CSF#
Chills and fever	−	+*
Bone pains	+*	+*
Extramedullary toxicities	+	+
Elevated LFTs	+	+
Cardiac toxicities	−	+*
Renal toxicities	−	+*
Pericardial toxicities	−	+*
Peripheral edema	−	+

#Information pertaining to either sargramostim or regramostim

*Dose-dependent toxicities (Occurring most frequently when doses are >15 µg/kg)

Adapted from Louie *et al.*

Table 7.6. Adverse effect profile of CSFs.

clinical adverse events, including alopecia, nausea, vomiting, diarrhea, mucositis, and myelosuppression. Common hematological toxicities consist primarily of anemia, thrombocytopenia, and neutropenia. However, the major consequence in patients with severe neutropenia, where the absolute neutrophil count (ANC) is below 500 cells/μL, is increased risk of developing life-threatening infections. Chronic or persistent suppression of white blood counts (WBC) above 1000 cell/μL may also predispose patients to opportunistic infections.

Since neutrophils play a critical role as a phagocytes against microbial invaders, it is not surprising that these patients are susceptible to bacterial, fungal, and other opportunistic infections. Although improvements in empirical antibiotic therapy have stemmed the mortality rate, only with amelioration of the immuncompromised condition can the patient hope to survive continual microbial assaults. Efforts to boost the immune system have included granulocyte transfusions into the immunocompromised patient. However, granulocyte transfusions have failed to show any significant benefits. Rather, granulocyte infusions were associated with higher rates of developing *de nova* cytomegalovirus infections, a life-threatening viral infection in the immunocompromised patient.

Chemotherapy-induced pancytopenia presents another problem, where prolonged neutropenia may result in delays to subsequent doses of chemotherapy. Patients who are unable to continue on the established protocols without either schedule delay or dosage attenuation seem to have a poorer outcome than patients who receive chemotherapy on schedule. Delays and dosage reductions have been arguably the central issue of controversy as to the effectiveness of certain protocols, especially those chemotherapy regimens containing myelosuppressive agents.

GRANULOCYTE-COLONY STIMULATING FACTOR

The effectiveness of recombinant G-CSF (rhG-CSF) was evaluated in patients with transitional cell carcinoma (TCCA) receiving cytoxic chemotherapy. During cycles where rhG-CSF was administered, all patients were able to receive their scheduled chemotherapy, whereas during cycles where rhG-CSF support was withdrawn, only 33% of the patients were able to receive their scheduled chemotherapy on time.

rhG-CSF was evaluated for its ability to accelerate neutrophil recovery, and prevent infections in small cell lung carcinoma (SCLC) patients. These patients were given a chemotherapy regimen consisting of cyclophosphamide, doxorubicin, and etoposide. Patients were randomized in a double-blinded fashion to receive either rhG-CSF or placebo. The median duration of severe neutropenia (<500 cells/mm³) in patients receiving rhG-CSF was significantly

shorter than paired controls. There was a reduction in the number of days where the neutrophils were below 500 neutrophils/mm³, correlating with a drop in neutropenic fever. This trend continued throughout the study, where a 37% reduction in neutropenic fever was evident in the group receiving rhG-CSF when compared to the paired controls. The reduced number of episodes of neutropenic fever was accompanied by a 47% reduction in antibiotic usage. The reduction in neutropenic fever also corresponded to a reduction in hospitalization.

GRANULOCYTE-MACROPHAGE COLONY STIMULATING FACTOR

GM-CSF has been studied in patients with advanced malignancies and sarcoma. Patients with advanced malignancies were given varying doses of GM-CSF at least four weeks after they had received their last chemotherapy or radiation treatment. Following initial administration of GM-CSF, a transient decrease in absolute neutrophil counts (ANC) persisted for approximately four hours followed by a dose-dependent rise. This rapid rise of neutrophils could be attributed to release of neutrophil progenitors, demarginalization of neutrophils from blood vessel walls, and prolonged neutrophil survival. There was no consistent effect on either hemoglobin levels or platelets counts in these patients. However, there was a dose-dependent increase in the number of circulating eosinophils and basophils when GM-CSF was given.

The effects of GM-CSF were studied in patients with metastatic or inoperable sarcoma. Because *in vitro* studies have shown that GM-CSF was able to stimulate tumor cell proliferation, GM-CSF was given to patients prior to the chemotherapy administration to evaluate if this cytokine could promote tumor proliferation. No tumor progression was seen in this study. Instead, it was found that pre-chemotherapy infusion of GM-CSF was able to increase circulating granulocytes in a dose-dependent manner. Following chemotherapy, GM-CSF (dosage ranging from 4–64 μg/kg/day) was administered as a continuous transfusion during the first cycle of chemotherapy.

Neutrophils and white blood counts (WBC) from the first cycle were compared to those found in the second cycle where GM-CSF support was withdrawn. A dose-dependent increase of WBC and ANC throughout the dosage ranges were seen in cycle one, when GM-CSF support was given. Although *in vitro* studies have shown that GM-CSF is able to increase megakaryocytes, no significant improvements in platelet recovery were seen. This may be due to a lower concentration of GM-CSF used as compared to *in vitro* studies.

When GM-CSF was given at 5 μg/kg/day to patients with SCLC patients who were treated with a chemotherapy regimen of etoposide and carboplatinum. The duration of the GM-CSF therapy was given either for 7, 14, or 21 days. Of the patients who received GM-CSF, 9% of patients experienced severe neutropenia (ANC<500 cell/µl). This is contrast to historical controls, where 38% of patients developed grade IV neutropenia. Results suggest that GM-CSF was also able to ameloriate both the duration and severity of neutropenia.

These results suggest that both G-CSF and GM-CSF are able to ameliorate chemotherapy-induced neutropenia. A reduction of neutropenic fever suggests that CSF stimulated cells are functional and are able to prevent opportunistic infections.

CSFs in Acquired Immunodeficiency Syndrome

Acquired immunodeficiency syndrome (AIDS) is a viral infection attacking the helper T4 lymphocyte (CD4⁺), which is the cornerstone of humoral and cellular regulation. A progressive drop in CD4⁺ cells will lead to immune system dysfunction, where cytokine expression is altered and cause a downregulation of cellular immunity. These changes place HIV infected patient at risk for opportunistic infections (see Chapter 6).

GRANULOCYTE-MACROPHAGE COLONY STIMULATING FACTOR

Although the most prominent clinical finding in AIDS is a decline in CD4⁺ cells, the immune responsiveness of myeloid cells is changed due to altered lymphocyte expression of cytokines as compared to non-HIV infected patients. When GM-CSF was given to patient with AIDS with leukopenia, a dose-dependent increase in circulating WBC was observed, especially peripheral neutrophils, eosinophils, and monocytes. In addition, GM-CSF was able to reverse neutrophil dysfunction. An increase in neutrophil activity, such as improved chemotaxis towards f-Met-Leu-Phe (agent use for in vitro assay for neutrophil chemotactic activity) and superoxide production (an indicator of cytotoxic activity), was seen after the initiation of GM-CSF therapy. When GM-CSF was given, there was an increase in circulating eosinophils that even exceeded the number of mature circulating neutrophils. Although a transient lymphocyte elevation was seen in a few patients, GM-CSF did not alter the T4/T8 ratio.

Patients with HIV often receive drugs that can affect bone marrow and prevent its ability to generate circulating cells (e.g. ganciclovir and cytotoxic chemotherapy). When GM-CSF was given to AIDS patients with cytomegalovirus (CMV), it was able to ameliorate ganciclovir-induced leukopenia. Subcutaneous injections of GM-CSF were given a dose range from 1 to 15 µg/kg/day. Patients receiving doses above 5 µg/kg/day were able to sustain ANC in the normal range, where peripheral leukocytes increased 50 to 90% above baseline levels. These results suggest that GM-CSF was able to mitigate myelosuppressive activity of antiviral agents like ganciclovir. Despite an increase in neutrophils, some patients experience an increase of serum p24 when GM-CSF was administered. The rise in p24 suggests that GM-CSF may activate HIV proliferation.

GM-CSF induced HIV proliferation was confirmed through an in vitro study where HIV-infected cells were incubated in the presence of various CSFs. Both class I CSF, IL-3 and GM-CSF, were able to increase p24. GM-CSF was able to stimulate the highest level of p24 in monocytes infected with HIV. M-CSF was also able to increase p24, but not at the levels seen with GM-CSF. In contrast, G-CSF had no effect on the p24 levels, which may be due to G-CSF's inability to activate the monotropic HIV cell line (HTLV IIIb). The mechanism of viral activation is attributed to the ability of IL-3 and GM-CSF to stimulate the long terminal repeat (LTR), the promoter of tat gene, which increases transcription of viral proteins.

Conversely, GM-CSF was able to increase the incorporation of zidovudine (AZT) into viral DNA. Increased AZT incorporation may increase the susceptibility of HIV to antiviral therapy, where inhibition of HIV replication was attributed to ability of GM-CSF to enhance intracellular phosphorylation of AZT in infected monocytes. In fact, the combination of GM-CSF with stavudine and zidovudine has been shown to be synergistic. However, when GM-CSF is combined with didanosine or zalcitabine, antagonism was demonstrated. When GM-CSF is used in HIV patients, antiretroviral agents should be used.

GRANULOCYTE-COLONY STIMULATING FACTOR

G-CSF has also been employed in patients with HIV. Similar to GM-CSF, G-CSF is able to elevate WBCs, especially neutrophils. G-CSF is able to restore neutrophil activity, where myeloperoxidase and chemotactic activity was significantly increased. Unlike GM-CSF, G-CSF did not increase p24 suggesting that it did not stimulate HIV replication. This was also confirmed in an in vitro study.

Patients with HIV seem to need less G-CSF, when compared to non-HIV patients, to achieve the same level of WBC. This is attributed to the high level of IL-1 in HIV patients, which can prime and mobilize G-CSF sensitive progenitor cells.

The effect of G-CSF and epoietin alfa was evaluated in AIDS and ARC patients, who were intolerant to antiviral agents, as evidenced by the development anemia and leukopenia. Following a four week washout period where myelosuppressive agents were discontinued, patients were started at 1.2 μg/kg/day of subcutaneously administered G-CSF. The addition of G-CSF was able to produced a significant increase in mean ANC as compared to baseline indices (p-value <0.05). After reaching targeted ANC, patients were then initiated on epoeitin alfa (150 units/kg) given three times a week. All patients were able to achieve or surpass the target hemoglobin levels within 5 weeks of therapy. In the fourth stage of this study, patients were restarted on zidovudine at 1,000 to 1,500 mg/day given orally in five divided doses. A dosage increase of 0.3 to 1.2 μg/kg/day was required to maintain the target ANC after AZT was reinstituted.

CSFs in HIV Malignancy

GM-CSF was also given to patients with AIDS associated NHL who were to receive a chemotherapy regimen containing cyclophosphamide, doxorubicin, vincristine, and prednisone (CHOP). Patients were randomized to one of three groups, where GM-CSF was given at 10–20 μg/kg/day either on days 1–10 or days 4–13, or no CSF support at all. No significant difference was seen in patients not receiving CSFs as compared to those receiving GM-CSF from days 1 to 10. However, patients treated on days 4–13 had a shorter duration of neutropenia as compared to the untreated group. Serum p24 levels were elevated, suggesting HIV replication, during the GM-CSF treatment period. The p24 level returned to baseline after cessation of GM-CSF. Although p24 was raised with GM-CSF, no clinical signs of HIV progression were noted.

AIDS patients with Kaposi's sarcoma can be treated with a combination of interferon-α (IFN-α) and AZT. Unfortunately, patients develop myelosuppression with long-term therapy. In one study, 19 of 29 patients developed neutropenia (<1000 cells/mm³), which required GM-CSF support. Patients receiving 125 μg/m²/day GM-CSF as a SC injection were shown to increase and sustain ANC.

G-CSF was also found to be effective in accelerating bone marrow recovery in HIV patients receiving cytotoxic chemotherapy for either NHL or Kaposi's Sarcoma. Bone marrow suppressive effects were ameliorated with G-CSF support, where the bone marrow recovery was similar to that seen with GM-CSF. Unlike some patients who received GM-CSF, there was no elevation of serum p24 in these patients.

Pathogenesis of Septic Shock

Septic shock is a leading cause of mortality in patients admitted to intensive care units. Over 100,000 patients die yearly of septic shock, despite the correct selection of antibiotics and vasopressor. This syndrome is initiated by the presence of bacteria in the circulation (bacteremia). Septic shock syndrome occurs most frequently during gram-negative bacteremia. Although septic shock may occur with gram-positive organisms such as *Staphylococcus aureus* (i.e. toxic shock syndrome), septic shock syndrome is more associated with lipopolysaccharides (LPS) on the surface of gram-negative organisms. LPS have been shown to be potent stimulators of immune activation. In fact, septic shock syndrome may be described as an exaggerated immune response to LPS resulting in overproduction of inflammatory mediators, such as TNF and IL-1. When an individual is in septic shock, massive quantities of TNF and IL-1 are produced.

IL-1 and TNF are endogenous pyrogens capable of inducing fever, chills, myalgias, and arthalgias. Fevers and flu-like symptoms may be further augmented by the ability of TNF and IL-1 to increase production of prostaglandins. Antipyretic agents such as acetaminophen, aspirin, and ibuprofen are able to reduce fever by blocking TNF and IL-1-mediated activities, but are unable to affect the expression of these pro-inflammatory mediators.

IL-1 and TNF mediated vascular injuries may result in increased capillary leakage, thus reducing intravascular volume, as evidenced by a drop in mean arterial pressure (MAP). The body will compensate for the drop in blood pressure by increasing the heart rate. A second deleterious effect of TNF is its ability to depress myocardial contractility, which can decrease the effectiveness of the compensatory heart rate increase. Furthermore, TNF is able to reduce blood pressure and tissue perfusion by relaxing vascular smooth muscle tone thus reducing systemic vascular resistance. This reduction of muscle tone can be mediated directly or indirectly by TNF-induced production of vasodilators, such as prostaglandins and nitric oxide. Organ perfusion can further be decreased by the TNF-mediated coagulation cascade and activation of neutrophil adhesion leading to vascular plugging. The drop in organ perfusion for an extended period can lead to irreversible organ damage, resulting in death.

IL-1 and TNF can cause vascular endothelial cells to exhibit leukocytes adhesion, initially for neutrophils and then for monocytes and lymphocytes. These actions contribute to accumulation of leukocytes at local sites of inflammation. Furthermore, TNF is able to stimulate macrophages to produce cytokines, including IL-1, IL-6, TNF (autocrinic factor), and IL-8. Other TNF effects include stimulation of vascular endothelial cells and fibroblasts to produce CSFs.

Immunotherapy for Septic Shock

Currently, there is no treatment for septic shock. Strategies to treat septic shock include the elimination of the enhanced immunoactivation. Thus the elimination of endotoxin or lipopolysaccharide (LPS) using anti-LPS antibodies may be able to prevent the onset of septic shock syndrome. Two monoclonal antibodies, E5 and HA1A, have been tested in humans with septic shock. Because these agents are still unapproved by for use, the only means to prevent certain death is supportive care.

Supportive care begins with hemodynamic support such as with fluid challenge. If fluid challenge is unable to reverse IL-1 and/or TNF-induced hypotension, the use of β-adrenergic agonists and vasopressors such as dopamine, dobutamine, epinephrine and phenylephrine may be necessary to adequately support blood pressure for organ perfusion. This can be monitored by normalizing laboratory values (i.e. liver function tests, serum creatinine, and cardiac ejection fraction).

Although aggressive support care may be important in the acute phase of the syndrome, the elimination of the LPS is critical in determining clinical outcome. This may be accomplished by using appropriate antibiotics which are active against the pathogen. However, this may be a "double-edged sword" whereby antibiotic-induced bacterial lysis can increase levels of LPS.

The use of steroids to blunt LPS-induced immunoactivation has been controversial in its ability to prevent, or even ameliorate septic shock syndrome. Other means, such as with naloxone, an antagonist of beta-endorphins and opioids, have been explored with limited clinical success. Therefore, current treatment relies on effective antibiotic coverage and aggressive supportive care.

Future therapeutic options will include the use of monoclonal antibodies directed against the antigen, LPS or inflammatory cytokines like IL-1 and TNF. Both murine (E5) and humanized (HA1A) monoclonal antibody is able to bind onto free LPS to prevent septic shock syndrome. However the window of clinical opportunity is narrow in that LPS immunostimulation may reach a point where elimination of circulating LPS will have no impact on the clinical outcome. Another therapeutic option is to inhibit the increase in primary inflammatory mediators, such as TNF and IL-1. A competitive antagonist of IL-1 or interleukin-1 receptor antagonist(IIL-1ra) has been shown to be safe and effective in ameliorating septic shock syndrome. IL-1ra is an analog of IL-1 that binds onto the IL-1 receptor but does not induce IL-1 biological activity. Preliminary results suggest that it is effective in patients with mild to moderate septic shock. Alternative strategies include monoclonal antibodies directed against TNF. Recently, soluble receptors have been isolated for cytokines such as TNF, IL-2, and IL-6. These cytokine "sponges" will bind onto the cytokines, thus reducing the levels of free proinflammatory cytokines for immune activation. Although the principle behind soluble receptors is sound, their use in the clinical setting has been disappointing.

Infectious Disease

The role of neutrophils and macrophages in the eradication of bacterial and fungal infections is well documented. CSFs play a critical role in mobilizing and recruiting these cellular elements to the sites of infections. CSFs has been shown to reverse alcohol and thermal-induced immunosuppression.

Foreign substances such as ethanol have been shown to inhibit both the humoral and the cellular response to bacterial infections. Alcohol represses the cellular response by inhibiting CSF production. Rats intoxicated with ethanol were unable to produce adequate amounts of TNF, which may explain the decreased number of polymorphonuclear cells found at the site of infection. The inability to mount a cellular response may contribute to the increased incidence of morbidity associated with infectious complications.

G-CSF was able to enhance the host defense in normal and ethanol-induced immunosuppressed rats that were infected with *Klebsiella pneumoniae*. Statistically significant improvement in survival was seen in ethanol intoxicated rats that were given both antimicrobial therapy and G-CSF as compared to paired controls. These results are now being evaluated in a phase III trial determining if G-CSF is able to accelerate recovery in patients with severe community acquired pneumonias. Preliminary studies suggest that G-CSF was able to preserve organ function.

Thermal Injury

After thermal injury patients develop a mark leukocytosis, which is followed by substantial fall in circulating neutrophils. This leukocytopenia may be attribute to a rise in suppressor T-lymphocytes approximately five to seven hours after injury. A drop in circulating granulocytes correlates with increased serum lactoferrin, a neutrophil product found in neutrophil granules. *In vitro* studies have found that lactoferrin was able to inhibit the production of G-CSF in freshly isolated mononuclear cells, which was reversed with the addition of exogenous G-CSF. G-CSF was combined with gentamicin in experimental thermal injury models. Mice with thermal injury seeded with *Pseudomonas aeruginosa* were given either G-CSF, gentamicin alone, or in combination together. Mice receiving the combination had significantly better survival as compared to both G-CSF and gentamicin alone, whereas all thermal injured mice that were untreated died within 8 days.

Mice sensitized with GalN were pre-treated with either GM-CSF or G-CSF. This was followed by lipopolysaccharide (LPS) administration one hour later. Mice treated with G-CSF were able to block LPS-induced TNF production when G-CSF was given 1 hour before or at the same time as LPS induction. There was no mortality in the groups given G-CSF prior to or simultaneously with LPS. When G-CSF was given 1 hour after LPS sensitization, no blunting of TNF was seen, which correlated with a 50% mortality. In contrast, when GM-CSF was given 1 hour before LPS administration, a 20 fold increase in TNF concentration was found, resulting in 80% mortality in the mice receiving this combination. This study suggests that GM-CSF may be synergistic with LPS to induce synthesis of TNF. Increased levels of TNF were correlated with a higher incidence of mortality. In contrast, pre-treatment with G-CSF was able to blunt LPS-induced expression of TNF.

These animal studies have provided some insight in the use of CSFs in the infection arena. Studies support the hypothesis that CSFs may be able to augment antibiotics in patients with bacterial infections and who may have immunosuppression. Furthermore, G-CSF has the ability to blunt LPS induction of TNF, whereas GM-CSF enhances TNF production. Thus, GM-CSF should be used cautiously in patients with documented gram-negative sepsis. ∎

References

- **Dexter TM, Moore M.** (1986). Growth and development in the hematopoietic system: the role of lymphockines and their possible therapeutic potential in disease and malignancies. *Carcinogenesis*, **7**, 509–516

- **Johnson GR, Keller GM, Nicola NA.** (1982). Differentiation and 'renewal' of multipotential cell *in vitro*. *J Cell Physiol.*, Suppl 1, 23–30

- **Louie SG, Jaresko GS.** (1991). Biological agents in infectious diseases. *J Pharm Pract.*, **5**, 326–341

- **Louie S, Jung B.** (1993). Clinical effects of biologic response modifiers. *Am J Hosp Pharm*, **50**, S10–18

- **Metcalf D.** (1989). The molecular control of cell division, differentiation commitment and maturation in haemopoietic cells. *Nature*, **339**, 27–30

- **Metcalf D.** (1988). Haemopoietic growth factors. *Therapeutics*, **148**, 516–519

- **Neumanatis J, Singer JW, Buckner CD,** *et al.* (1990). Use of recombinant human granulocyte macrophage colony stimulating factor in graft failure after bone marrow transplantation. *Blood*, **76**, 245–253

- **Oppenheim JJ, Ruscetti FW, Faltynek C.** (1994). Cytokines. In *Basic and Clinical Immunology Eight Edition*, edited by DP Stites, AI Terr, TG Parslow. Norwalk, Connecticut: Appleton & Lange, pp. 105–123

- **Sheridan WP, Bagley CG, Juttner CA,** *et al.* (1992). Effect of peripherial blood progenitor cells mobilised by filgrastim (G-CSF) on platelet recovery after high dose of chemotherapy. *Lancet*, 640–644

Case Study with Self-Assessment Questions

JQ is a 26 year old white male who had experienced 3 days of chills and fever. Four days prior to admission, he consumed two pints of whiskey along with 2 six-packs of beers. He developed nausea and vomited at least three times, before becoming unconscious. He was found unconscious by his room-mate the next morning. JQ had a "hangover" the next morning and began experiencing chest pain. His chest pains were compounded by difficulty breathing, which was exacerbated when he tried to walk upstairs. Symptoms worsened and were accompanied by high fevers, which prompted his room-mate to bring him into the emergency room. His admitting diagnosis was for aspiration pneumonia and possible bacteremia.

Social History   Ethanol consumption: at least a 6-pack a day.
                  Tobacco: 2 packs daily.

Laboratory:

Na	137(135–145)	Cl	106(101–111)	BUN	85(7–22)	Glu	102(70–110)
K	3.5(3.5–5.0)	CO_2	20.2(24–32)	Scr	3.6 (0.7–1.3)		
Ca	8.2 (8.2–10.6)	PO_4	3.2 (2.5–4.5)	Mg	1.8 (1.7–2.5)		
TPro	5.1 (6.0–8.0)	Alb	3.2 (3.2–5.5)	Tbili	1.7 (0.0–1.3)		
AP	119 (20–100)	AST	450 (5–40)	ALT	323 (5–40)		
LDH	82 (100–250)	UA	4.5 (3.5–7.2)				
WBC	20.7(4.1–10.9)	Hgb	13.4(13–16)	Hct	40.1(40–50)	Plt	110 (200–350)

X-ray: Left lower lobe consolidation consistent with aspiration pneumonia.

Sputum: Gram negative rods with gram positive cocci, with a few epithelial cells and many WBC

Culture: Blood: Pending.
              Sputum: Pending.

Vital Signs: Heart Rate : 104 beats/min   Respiratory Rate: 26 breaths/min
             Temperature: 39.1°C   Bp: 95/55 mm Hg

Question 1:   *What cytokine may be responsible for his vital sign changes? What is the biological activity of these cytokines?*

Question 2:   *If this patient is in septic shock, what intervention would you suggest? Give two immunotherapeutic options to treat septic shock.*

Answer 1:   Elevation of interleukin-1 and TNF is expected in these individuals. These two cytokines have pyrogenic effects. Which will cause fever, chills, rigors, hypotension?

Answer 2:   If the patient is in septic shock, levels of interleukin-1 and tumor necrosis factor (TNF-α) are elevated. These cytokines are responsible for the various biological activity which include high fever and drop in blood pressure. To compensate for vascular dilation, the heart rate is increased to maintain blood pressure. Blockade of both interleukin-1 and TNF may ameliorate fever, tachycardia, and hypotension. This can be accomplished through administration of monoclonal antibody directed against both cytokines. Alternatively, using an interleukin-1 receptor antagonist, a naturally occurring interleukin-1-like protein devoid of inflammatory activity, may block IL-1 mediated activity.

8 | Transplantation

Introduction

Organ transplantation has become an important modality in various types of disorders. Although the types of organ and cell transplantation have expanded (Table 8.1), the major obstacle confronting all organ transplantations continues to be graft rejection. This is where the immune system responds to the transplanted organ as if it was a foreign antigen, thus mounting an immunological attack. Like the response to any antigen, graft rejection is an immunological process where both humoral and cellular responses are required to orchestrate the defense.

Unlike the normal immune response against a foreign antigen or pathogen, the immunological response to a transplanted organ (allograft) is not a desirable effect. Thus, the objective in organ transplantation is to selectively suppress the immune activities directed against the allograft. However, a delicate balance must be employed to allow the desired immunological responses to continue to function normally. This is the challenge confronting organ transplantation, that is, to inhibit specific immune activation, while maintaining the anti-infective immune response.

With the advent of selective immunosuppressive agents, transplantations of organ, tissues, and bone marrow cells that were once considered as experimental procedures are now advanced as therapeutic options. As described above,

Types of transplantation
Heart
Kidney
Liver
Lung
Pancreas
Retina
Bone marrow

Table 8.1. Types of transplantation.

following transplantation of either allografts or allogeneic cells, the immune system of the recipient must be adequately and selectively suppressed to prevent graft rejection. Unlike organ transplantation, bone marrow transplantation (BMT) is the transfer of immunocompetent cells into the recipient. In this situation, the donor cells must be suppressed to prevent the engrafted cells from attacking host tissues, more commonly referred to as graft versus host disease (GvHD).

Types of Rejection

Transplant patients who are experiencing either organ rejection or graft versus host disease (GvHD) may have some of the following signs and symptoms. Signs may include swelling and tenderness at or near the site of organ transplantation. Systemic symptoms may include chills, fever, malaise, cachexia, and generalized myalgias. Laboratory signs may also include elevation of circulating white blood cells (WBCs), lymphocyte infiltration into the allograft, elevated liver enzymes, and serum creatinine. Elevated markers of liver function tests like aminotransferases and alkaline phosphatase, may indicated hepatocyte destruction in liver transplant recipients. Renal transplant recipients experiencing increased serum creatinine could indicate rejection of the transplanted kidney.

Organ rejection can be subclassified into various types. There are three types of graft rejection which are as follows: hyperacute, acute, and chronic graft rejection. The type of rejection is defined by the timing after the allograft transplantation, and the immune response that is associated with the rejection process. Hyperacute rejection is usually attributed to pre-existing antibodies directed against red blood cells (RBCs), which shares surface antigens with endothelial cells that line the walls of the vasculature. In contrast, acute and chronic rejection is associated with lymphocytes that are directed against the graft itself.

Hyperacute Graft Rejection

Hyperacute graft rejection is humoral mediated rejection where the recipient has pre-formed antibodies directed against the surface antigens on the donor's RBCs. These antibodies are also referred to as ABO isohemagglutinins, and are cross-reactive to endothelial cells surface antigen. ABO isohemagglutinins binding onto vascular endothelium will trigger an immune cascade directed against the vasculature. Initially, complement fixation will occur, which is followed by cellular activation. In addition, the deposition of IgG onto the endothelial cells will activate antibody dependent cell-mediated cytotoxicity (ADCC) against the endothelial cells. In response to tissue injury, the body will activate the clotting pathways to prevent additional intravascular loss. These events can result in microthrombi formation within capillary loops and arterioles. When enough of the capillaries are occluded, severe ischemia and necrosis of the graft can occur.

Clinical management of hyperacute rejection includes antiplatelet and anticoagulant therapy to reduce the number of capillaries occluded, and restore perfusion to the allograft. At present, there are no effective means of treating these type of lesions. Therefore, emphasis must be placed on careful tissue and blood typing to assess the degree of donor specific sensitization to HLA antigens using cross-matching tests. Other preemptive measures include minimizing the number of blood transfusions which may sensitize recipients to alloantigens, thus increasing the risk of hyperacute rejections.

Acute Graft Rejection

The most commonly encountered rejection is acute graft rejection. This type of rejection is mediated by antigen presenting cells (APC) such as macrophages, Kupffer cells, and dentritic cells. The molecular mechanism of this process is initiated by the release of antigens by the allograft, which are taken up and processed by APCs. The processed antigen is presented to dormant CD4+ cells along with MHC class II antigen. Immune activation occurs when antigen presentation occurs through co-stimulation with cytokine stimulus.

Antigen presentation along with cytokine co-stimulating with either IL-1 or TNF will activate dormant CD4+ cells to produce IL-2, which will modulate cellular immunity. Elevation of IL-2 will amplify and expand both CD4 and CD8 effector cells that will directly induce the anti-graft responses. CD4 mediated cellular cytotoxicity is similar to type IV or delayed-type hypersensitivity (DTH) reaction, where CD4 cells can recognize cells bearing HLA-DR surface antigen. CD4 cytotoxic activity is unlike the CD8 mediated activity, which is focused on cells that have HLA-A and HLA-B antigens on their cellular membranes. In contrast, CD8-mediated cellular immunity occurs with expansion of CTL and NK cells which have infiltrated into allograft tissues.

Transplant patients who are experiencing acute graft rejection often have elevated levels of cytokines, such as IL-2, TNF, IL-1 and IFN-γ. IFN-γ can induce the expression of HLA-A, -B, and -DR on allograft tissues, and thereby increase graft vulnerability to cellular cytotoxic attacks. IFN-γ can also activate and enhance DTH responses. Moreover, IFN-γ in combination with IL-2 has synergistic activity that will enhance CD8-mediated cellular cytotoxicity.

Clinically, acute rejection is treated by escalating the dose of corticosteroids, which will reduce expression of monokines, and inhibit alloactivation of T-cells. These events will reduce IL-2 expression and downregulate the immune system. Despite using high doses of corticosteroids, acute graft rejection may still persist. When rejection is resistant to corticosteroid therapy, the use of antibody therapy is warranted. Anti-lymphocyte globulin (ALG) and OKT3 are commonly used in these types of situation, where cells bearing CD3 receptors are eliminated. If graft perfusion continues to deteriorate, removal of the graft may be necessary. Thus aggressive and prompt use of immunosuppressants is vital in preserving the allograft.

Chronic Graft Rejection

This type of rejection has a slow onset and may occur months to years following the initial transplantation. Chronic rejection process is characterized by narrowing of the arterial lumen (Figure 8.1). The pathological findings in a patient experiencing chronic graft rejection are similar to those seen in patients with coronary artery disease. In chronic rejection, vascular endothelial cells proliferate beyond the vascular bed and begin proliferating as multiple-cell layers. Overgrowth of endothelial cells will reduce the diameter of the vessel lumen and reduce blood flow to the affected area.

Though the exact mechanism of action is still unclear, there is evidence suggesting that this is an IL-1 mediated event. IL-1 can activate endothelial cells to release platelet-derived growth factor (PDGF), which can further promote endothelial cell proliferation. If this process is recognized early, it may be reversed using immunosuppressive therapy. However if it has progressed to the stage where fibrosis has occurred, the chronic rejection syndrome will be unresponsive to immunosuppressive therapy.

Graft Versus Host Disease

The use of bone marrow transplantation (BMT) for acute lymphoblastic leukemia (ALL), acute myelogous leukemia (AML), lymphomas, solid tumors, or other hematological disorders in patients is now a routine procedure. BMT is classified according to where the donor bone marrow is derived. Syngeneic and allogeneic BMT are from marrow

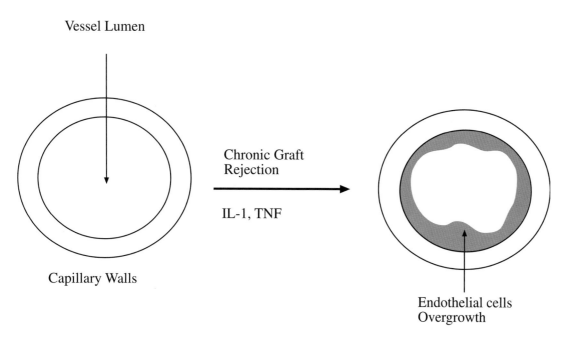

Vessel Lumen

Chronic Graft
Rejection

IL-1, TNF

Capillary Walls

Endothelial cells
Overgrowth

Figure 8.1. In chronic graft rejection, the lumen of capillaries supplying blood to the transplanted organ will narrow compared to pre-transplant status. The process is mediated by increased levels of inflammatory cytokines such as interleukin-1, which can induce platelet derived growth factor (PDGF) expression. These cytokines can increase endothelial cell proliferation, leading the cells to grow on top of each other and thus cause narrowing of the capillary lumen.

procured from either genetically identical twins or human leukocyte antigen (HLA)-matched individuals, respectively (Figure 8.2). In autologous BMT, the donor and recipient is the same individual, therefore no rejection is anticipated. The major difference between the various BMT is the degree of GvHD, which is dependent on the level of immunological compatibility or histocompatibility. This is similar to organ rejection, where the immune system mounts an attack on tissues which it recognizes as foreign; however, the difference between GvHD versus organ rejection is that the transplanted marrow attacks the recipient host.

In autologous BMT, GvHD is rarely if ever encountered because donor and host are identical. The same observation may be seen in syngeneic BMT; however, syngeneic GvHD occurs more frequently than in autologous BMT. Despite the fact that allogeneic BMT are normally HLA-matched, the histocompatibility between the donor and recipient is not complete because this test only compares major antigens on the surface of leukocytes and not all the tissues found in the body. Therefore, even when complete HLA-matching is accomplished, patients receiving allogeneic BMT will encounter some degree of GvHD.

In GvHD, the graft will begin to mount an attack on the host's tissue, recognizing the host's surface antigens as foreign, therefore giving rise to "graft versus host." GvHD is a life threatening immunological disease which primarily involves the gastrointestinal (GI) tract, skin, and liver.

Clinical presentation of GvHD may include high fever, rashes, and diarrhea. Laboratory findings may include an elevated liver function test (LFT) such as lactate dehydrogenase (LDH), alkaline phosphatase (AP), and bilirubin (bili). GvHD occurs in 100% of patients receiving allogeneic bone marrow transplant (BMT); however the severity or grading differs from patient to patient (Table 8.2). The severity is dependent on the degree of ABO and MHC incompatibilities.

Three immunological conditions must exist for GvHD to occur. These conditions include 1) immunological competence of the transplanted graft; 2) the presence of immunogenic antigen on the host tissues; 3) host inability to mount immunological reactions against the graft. Animals receiving allogeneic bone marrow transplantation will

Type of BMT	Marrow Donor	Risk of GvHD
Allogeneic BMT	HLA-matched sibling or donor	High
Syngeneic BMT	HLA-identical twin	Low
Autologous BMT	Self	Low

Table 8.2. Types of bone marrow transplantation.

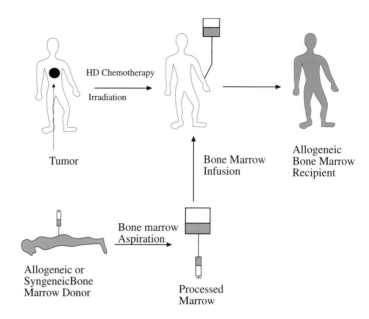

Allogeneic Bone Marrow Transplantation

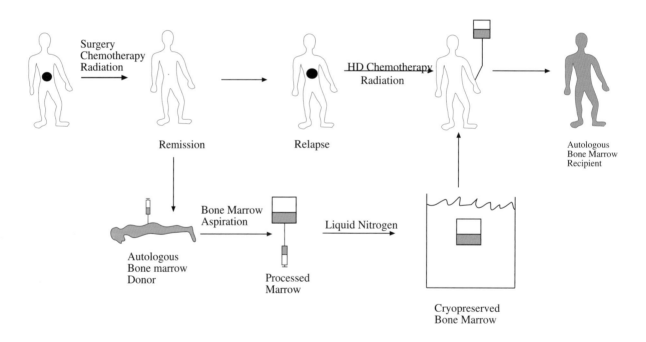

Autologous Bone Marrow Transplantation

Figure 8.2. There are various types of BMT, determined by the source of donor marrow. Allogeneic and syngeneic BMT are bone marrow derived from HLA-matched siblings or identical twin, respectively. In autologous BMT, the bone marrow and the recipient are the same individual. (A) Allogeneic or syngeneic donors marrow harvested, processed, and infused into the recipients. (B) Patients with tumors are treated with surgery, chemotherapy, and/or radiation, and their bone marrow is harvested. The processed marrow is cryopreserved in liquid nitrogen until the patient develops relapse disease. Prior to bone marrow infusion, the recipients existing bone marrow is cytoreduced using high dose chemotherapy and/or total body irradiation.

Grade	Skin	Liver	Gut
I	Epidermal basal cell vacuolar degeneration.	<25% small interlobular bile ducts abnormal	Single-cell necrosis of epithelial cells
II	Grade I changes plus "eosinophilic bodies"	25–50% bile ducts abnormal	Necrosis and dropout of glands
III	Grade II changes plus separation of the dermis	50–75% bile ducts	Focal microscopic glands and mucosal denudation
IV	Frank epidermal denudation	>75% bile ducts	Diffuse mucous necrosis

Table 8.3. Signs and symptoms of GVHD.

develop erythroderma, diarrhea, and jaundice if immuno-suppressants are not employed. Progression of these clinical symptoms will ultimately result in death. Skin biopsy from these recipients shows vacuolar alteration of the basilar epidermis and dyskeratoic epithelial cells in the epidermis or hair follicles. Advanced disease will manifest as frank subepidermal bulla formation (Table 8.3). Lymphocytic infiltration and necrosis of the bile ducts are hallmarks in skin and liver biopsies of allogeneic BMT recipients. Denudation of the intestinal tract is evident, which may explain severe diarrhea.

Lymphocytic infiltration into the tissues was initially identified as T-cells, juxtaposed to dying or necrotic cells. However, immunohistochemical studies identified that the majority of effector cells found in the tissues were natural killer cells (NKC) rather than cytotoxic T-lymphocytes. This led to the conclusion that GvHD is a NKC and not CTL mediated attack on host cells. However the controversy as to the exact cellular mechanism of GvHD is yet to be resolved.

Transplantation Immunology

The major objective in transplant immunology is to permit the transplanted organ or allograft to survive and function normally in the recipient. It is the presence of foreign antigens found on the surface of transplanted tissues that invokes the rejection process.

In order to develop anti-rejection strategies, it is essential to understand immunological compatibility or "histocompatibility." Tissue compatibility between the donor and the recipients is essential in reducing the potential of rejection. There a number of factors that can reduce the likelihood of graft rejection. This includes compatibility of blood and tissue type. As described in Chapter 5, red blood cells have antigens on their cellular membranes which are referred to as A, B, and O serotypes. Incompatibility of

ABO serotypes can lead to hyperacute rejection. The mismatch of the major histocompatibility complex (MHC) can lead to acute rejection. MHC matched organ transplantations have lower risk of developing graft rejection. The degree of difference or incompatibility in the cell surface antigens between donor and recipient can determine the timing and intensity of the rejection process.

MHC is a crucial component for recognition that can activate the immune cascade. Other important biological activities involving MHC include induction of humoral response, B-cell activation, and T-cell stimulation in response to viral infection and organ transplantation. These antigenic complexes allow the body to differentiate between "self and non-self." The importance of MHC in transplant immunology is its role in antigen recognition by cytotoxic T-lymphocytes (CTL) and natural killer (NK) cells, which are the primary effector cells responsible for graft rejection.

In humans, MHC is often referred to as human leukocyte antigen or HLA, where the HLA genes are closely clustered together on the short arm of chromosome 6 (Figure 8.3). There are two major classes of transplant antigens and they are referred to as Class I and II. The expression of Class I HLA antigen is regulated by HLA-A, HLA-B, and HLA-C genes. These antigens are found on the surface of virtually every cell, except red blood cells and embryonic cells. Cytotoxic T-lymphocytes (CTLs) have receptor Class I antigens, which use these antigens to "home in and anchor" onto the target cells to exert this cytotoxic activity.

In contrast, the expression of Class II antigen is regulated by HLA-D that has at three genes, designated as HLA-DR, -DQ, and -DW loci. The cells bearing Class II MHC antigens are restricted to antigen presenting cells (i.e. macrophage, Kupffer cells, and dentritic) and activated T-lymphocytes. They are important for antigen presentation to T-helper lymphocytes which have the Class II MHC receptors. Increased expression of Class II antigen can occur after interferon-γ activation.

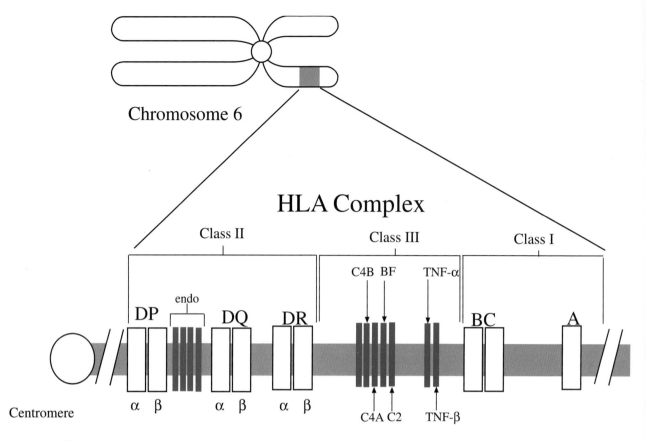

Figure 8.3. The major histocompatibility complex (MHC) or human leukocyte antigen (HLA) is located on the short arm of the sixth chromosome. This region contains the coding sequence of three classes of MHC proteins. In addition, this complex contains the encoding regions for complement factors (e.g. C2, C4, B, and F) and tumor necrosis factors α and β.

T-Cell Activation

The cellular component of the immune system mediates both graft rejections and GvHD. CD3/T-cell receptor (TCR) complex on the T-lymphocytes recognizes antigens by binding onto the peptide within the grooves formed by the MHC proteins. Activation of the T-lymphocyte is a result of cellular recognition of a foreign antigen that is present on allograft tissues. Following T-cell activation, there is a series of transcriptional signals leading to expression of lymphokines and their receptors, which will provide the growth stimulus (mitogenic) for CD4 and CD8 cell expansion (Figure 8.4). Activated CD4 cells produce and secrete lymphokines that will lead to both natural killer cell and cytotoxic T-lymphocyte activation, which ultimately mediates cellular attack on allograft tissues.

Antigen binding onto the CD3/TCR alone is not significant to activate the immune system (Figure 8.4). There must be a co-stimulation with inflammatory cytokines, such as IL-1 and TNF. Antigen binding and cytokine co-stimulation will activate a series of intracellular signals. These cytosolic signal pathways involve a number of biochemical intermediates that terminate with the transcription of

lymphokine and their receptors. Cellular expansion and activation is dependent on IL-2 secretion and the expression of IL-2 receptor (IL-2R) on the effector cells.

There are two major signal tranduction pathways that lead to transcription of lymphokines resulting in immuno-activation. One of these pathways is related to the activation of *ras*. The other pathway is calcium-dependent (Ca²⁺-dependent) phosphorylation of serine/threonine. The blockade of these intracellular signals or signal transduction can inhibit IL-2 and IL-2R transcription (Figure 8.5).

A number of pharmaceutical agents have been isolated to block these intracellular signals, including cyclosporine and FK506. Both of these agents are able to interrupt the Ca²⁺-dependent pathway. Cyclosporine (CSA) is a cyclic undecapeptide, whereas FK506 is a macrolide lactone. Despite being structurally different, both of these agents are capable of inhibiting lymphokine transcription such as IL-2, IL-3, IL-4, TNF, and GM-CSF, by terminating the same transduction signal. These immunosuppressive agents bind onto intracellular receptors called immunophilin receptors. Cytosolic receptors that bind onto FK506 are called FK binding proteins (FKBP), whereas cyclosporine binding proteins are referred to as cyclophilins. Though

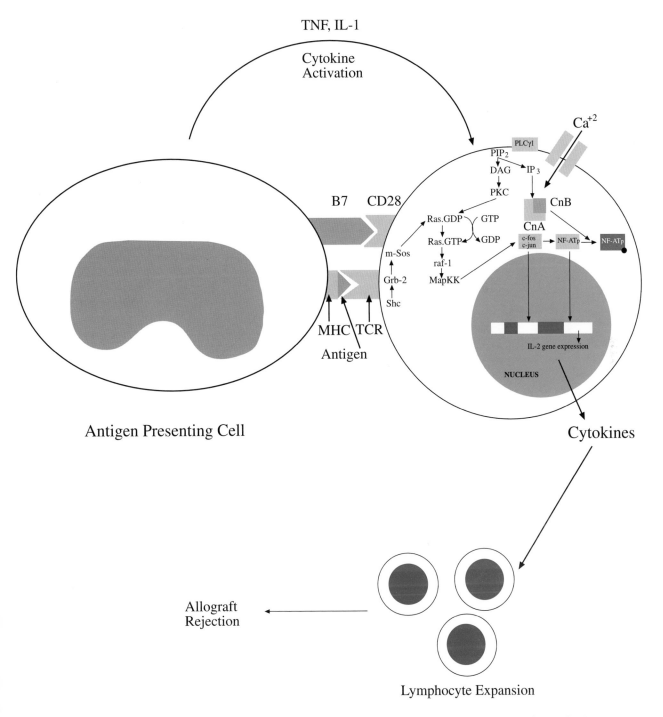

Figure 8.4. Following T-cell activation via antigen presentation and co-stimulation with either B7 or cytokines, there is a series of transcriptional signals leading to expression of lymphokines and their receptors. The expression of IL-2 will expand the population of T-lymphocytes which may result in activate graft rejection.

the two types of receptors differ in structure, they both have peptidyl-prolyl cis-trans isomerase (PPIase) activity which promotes immunoactivation. The blockade of PPIase activity can inhibit IL-2 expression thus blocking T-cell activation.

ABO Blood Types

As described in Chapter 5, ABO is a set of antigens that are found on the surfaces of red blood cells (RBCs) and vascular endothelial cells. Incompatiblity in ABO antigens

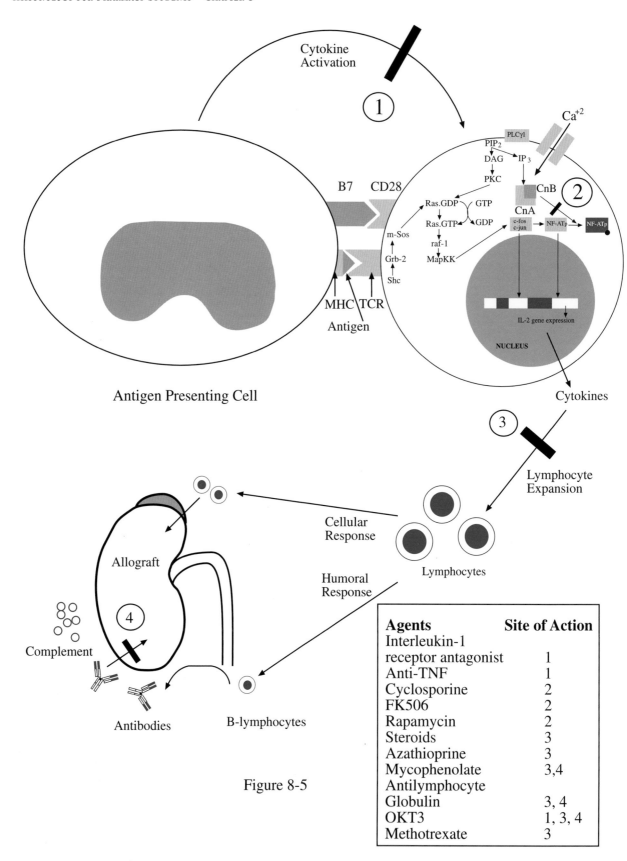

Antigen Presenting Cell

Figure 8-5

Agents	Site of Action
Interleukin-1 receptor antagonist	1
Anti-TNF	1
Cyclosporine	2
FK506	2
Rapamycin	2
Steroids	3
Azathioprine	3
Mycophenolate	3,4
Antilymphocyte Globulin	3, 4
OKT3	1, 3, 4
Methotrexate	3

Figure 8.5. The pharmacological mechanisms of action of various anti-graft rejection agents are detailed in this diagram.

between donor and recipient can cause rapid graft rejection that is initiated by isohemagglutinin-mediated vascular endothelium injury. In response to vascular damage, the clotting cascade will form microthrombi to prevent intravascular leakage. Although the microthrombus is initially beneficial to prevent additional intravascular leakage, the clot formation can also reduce blood flow to the transplanted organ. Prolonged reduction of blood flow causes oxygen starvation and can lead to tissue ischemia, which ultimately results in graft failure.

To alleviate the risk of anti-ABO mediated rejection or hyperacute rejection, ABO matching between donor and recipient is crucial. Complete ABO matching is not always available; in this situation partial ABO matching may be necessary. In these cases, recipients with AB blood type can receive grafts from donors with A, B, or O. Patients with type O antigen can donate to recipients with AB, A, B, or O serotypes with minimum antibody development. However, the optimal condition is to match each serotype with their own respective serotype.

One clinical measure to manage ABO incompatibility is to eliminate anti-ABO antibodies by removing the plasma of the recipient. This can be accomplished through a process called plasma exchange or plasmapheresis, where the patient's plasma is removed by a centrifugation process. Following plasma removal, fresh frozen plasma or albumin is used to replace the removed plasma. Anti-ABO antibodies can also be reduced by administrating cyclophosphamide (CTX) which inhibits B-cell expansion and antibody production. However, the long-term safety and efficacy of these methods have not been proven, and the utilization of these procedures may thus be limited.

Laboratory Tests for Compatibility

ABO matching has been established in the prevention of hyperacute rejection. In addition, there is compelling evidence correlating acute graft rejection with tissue MHC incompatibility. Laboratory tests to cross-match tissues between donors and recipients are vital. Matching HLA antigens or tissue typing can be accomplished through laboratory methods that include homozygous typing cells (HTC testing) and the mixed lymphocyte culture (MLC) test for HLA compatibility.

In order to determine the degree of histocompatiblity, it is important to assess both the presence or activity of antibodies and cellular cytotoxicity activity between the donor and recipient lymphocytes. To assess the presence of antibodies directed against the donor tissues, serological testing is used, more commonly known as "Cross-matching." Cellular matching is determined by direct cell-mediated cellular lysis (CML) assays.

SEROLOGICAL METHODS IN HISTOCOMPATIBILITY TESTING

The purpose of cross-matching is to determine the presence of a recipient's antibodies directed against donor tissues. The presence of antibodies directed against donor tissue will indicate that the recipient has been sensitized to antigens present on the donor's tissues. Antibodies directed against the donor tissue suggest that the recipient has the ability to activate complement factors and cellular components resulting in graft rejection.

Complement-mediated cytotoxicity can lead to tissue injury and activate platelet aggregation. Platelet aggregation will activate coagulation factor to form fibrin clots. In addition to repairing injured tissues, clot formation also occludes the affected tissues, thus reducing blood flow to the affected area. This reduction in blood flow can lead to tissue infarct resulting in ischemia and thereby allograft failure.

CROSS MATCHING BY CELLULAR MEDIATED LYSIS

Acute graft rejection is primarily mediated by cellular cytotoxicity. Pathological examination of affected tissues will reveal lymphocyte infiltration. Closer analysis of these immune cells suggests that there is both cytotoxic T-lymphocytes as well as natural killer cells. The presence of these cells in the rejected organs suggests that these cells play an important role in acute graft rejection. Thus it is important to determine if the recipient's CTLs are sensitized to the donor tissues. CTLs mediate their cellular toxic activity via direct binding onto the target cells, followed by the formation of perforin complex on the surface of the target cells (Figure 8.6).

Mixed lymphocyte cytotoxicity (MLC) is used to determine the ability of recipient cells to react with antigens found on donor blood cells. This can be accomplished by labeling the targeted cell with a radioactive label such as chromium^{51} (or ^{51}Cr). Cells are incubated in medium containing the ^{51}Cr. After a period of incubation, non-incorporated label is washed off by centrifuging the cell mix then removing the cell-free solution. These radiolabeled target cells are then added into a culture containing the lymphocytes from the recipient's blood. After the cells are allowed to react for a defined period, the cell mixture is centrifuged to separate the medium from the cells. The amount of radioactivity in the cell-free medium is then determined. The presence of radioactivity in the cell-free medium suggests that lymphocytes from the recipient are able to cause cell lysis, thus indicating that the recipient is able to attack donor tissues. The amount of ^{51}Cr in the cell-free medium is a measurement

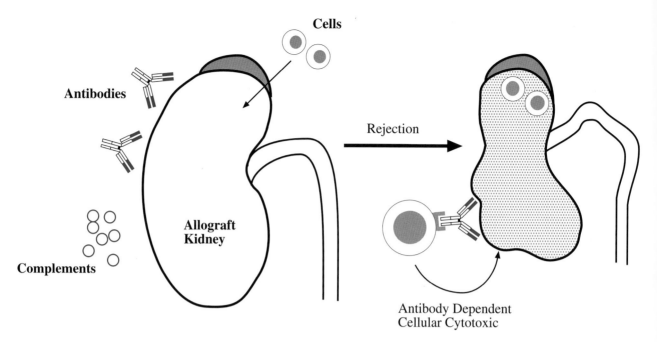

Figure 8.6. The mechanism of cellular-mediated graft rejection is detailed in this diagram. CTLs mediate their cellular toxic activity by direct binding onto the target cells. Following CTL binding onto the allograft, other immune responses which include antibody-dependent cellular cytotoxicity also occur.

of the recipient lymphocyte's ability to cause cellular donor tissues.

Immunosuppressive Agents
Corticosteroids

Steroid hormones are analogs of cholesterol consisting of four connecting five- or six-member rings. These agents, more specifically glucocorticoids or corticosteroids, are widely used as antiinflammatory agents. Clear-cut differentiation between antiinflammatory and immunosuppressive activities is not easy to distinguish. In addition, corticosteroids have anti-lymphocyte properties, and can induce programmed-cell death or "Apoptosis." Apoptosis is the activation of intracellular signals that leads to cellular breakdown without cellular lysis. The ability of corticosteroids to induce apoptosis in lymphocytes may account for their use in acute lymphoblastic leukemia (ALL) and lymphomas. Antiinflammatory and immunosuppressive activities can be classified into three categories, inhibition of circulatory activity, alteration of cellular functions, and antiinflammatory activity.

Corticosteroids have multiple effects on the immune system that include inhibition of lymphocyte clonal expansion through the blockade of expression of IL-1 and IL-2. In addition, steroids have antiinflammatory activity, which may contribute to the inhibition of lymphocyte prolifera-

tion. The molecular pharmacology of corticosteroids is thought to be production of antiinflammatory proteins and inhibiting the expression of proinflammatory cytokines (Figure 8.7).

Once steroids have transversed the cellular membrane, they bind onto a cytosolic receptor. This cytoplasmic receptor-steroid complex can also serve as a ligand for interphase nuclear receptors, where the binding of the receptor-steroid complex onto nuclear receptors regulates transcription of particular genes. The transcription of glycoproteins like lipomodulin is increased after exposure to corticosteroids. Lipomodulin is a phospholipase A2 inhibitor that can reduce the levels of arachidonic acid and its metabolites, the prostaglandins and leukotrienes that are mediators of tissue injury.

Other effects of corticosteroids include mobilization of neutrophils into the circulation as a result of steroid-induced demarginalization from the intravascular walls. Neutrophils that have been exposed to steroids have a reduced phagocytic activity, release degradative enzymes, and produce proinflammatory cytokines. So, despite the presence of more circulating neutrophils, there is a distinct decrease in neutrophil mediated activity.

In contrast to the initial neutrophilia seen following corticosteroid administration, there is a marked decline of circulating lymphocytes over time. The number of circulating B-cells or null cells is not significantly reduced. However, a marked decline in T-cells is found , more specifically

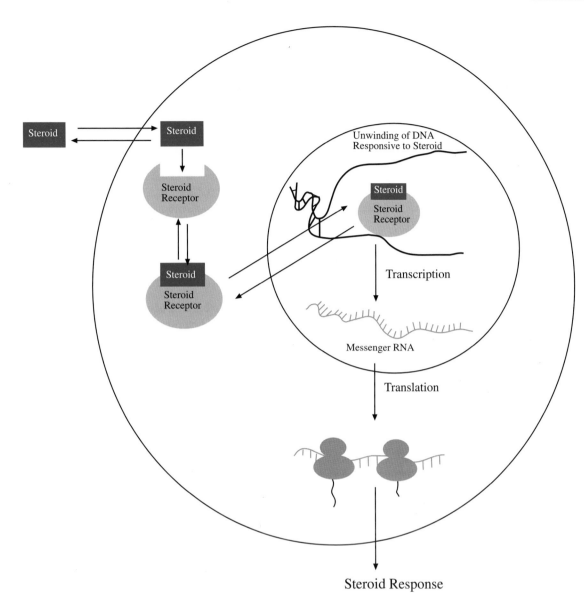

Figure 8.7. The molecular pharmacology of corticosteroids is thought to be production of anti-inflammatory proteins and inhibition of the expression of proinflammatory cytokines.

CD4 T-lymphocytes. Steroid-induced inhibition of IL-2 synthesis and secretion has been proposed as the primary mechanism for reduction of T-cell expansion. No changes in expression of IL-2 receptors or fall in IFN-γ level are apparent. This would suggest that the reduction of IL-2 is not based on a fall in IL-I mediated activities.

Other steroid-induced changes include a profound decline in monocytes. Monocyte/macrophage phagocytic activity is also impaired in the presence of steroids. Furthermore, macrophages exposed to corticosteroids have reduced Fc and complement receptors, thus reducing the ability for antigen recognition, processing and presentation. Steroids appear to exert their effects by preventing both the onset of chronic and acute immune responses.

Cytotoxic Agents

In graft rejection, cellular expansion is required to mount an immunological response to the allograft. Cytotoxic agents are primarily agents that interfere with cell cycling, preventing cells from entering G_o to G_I phase. The majority of these agents attempt to interfere with either the metabolism or nucleotide synthesis prior to cell cycling. There are two classes of cytotoxic agents that are used in the prevention of graft rejection: antimetabolites and nucleoside analogs.

A major problem associated with using cytotoxic agents in graft rejections is specificity. Rapidly growing cells will preferentially take up these agents, where cellular expansion requires DNA duplication for mitosis and meiosis. However, there are other cells which have a high turnover rate, such as blood cells, hair, and epithelial cells found in the gastrointestinal tract. The inability to selectively inhibit only lymphocytes leads to adverse effects such as myelo-suppression, gastrointestinal disturbance and alopecia.

Cytotoxic agents are rarely used as a single anti-rejection agents because they do not provide sufficient immuno-suppression to prevent the emergence of rejection. In con-trast, where higher doses of cytotoxic drugs are employed, unacceptable adverse effects may arise. Thus, they are primarily used in combination with corticosteroids, immuno-philin, binding agents or combination of both.

AZATHIOPRINES

Azathioprine is a prodrug where biotransformation of this agent is required to produce the active metabolite, 6-mercaptopurine (6MP). 6MP is a chemotherapeutic agent that is used in the treatment of lymphoblastic leukemia through termination of DNA synthesis. This inhibition of nucleic acid synthesis will prevent lymphocyte prolifera-tion and expansion, because purine analogs are preferen-tially taken up by lymphocytes.

CYCLOPHOSPHAMIDE

Cyclophosphamide (CTX) is an alkylating agent that is similar to azathioprine in that it requires hepatic metabo-lism to form the activity metabolite. Cyclophosphamide must be hydroxylated on the 4-position to form 4-hydroxycyclophosphamide (4HC). 4HC will undergo spon-taneous chemical reaction to form two metabolites, acrolein and phosphamide. Phosphamide, the active metabolite, can form covalent bonds between unwinding DNA strands, thus intercalating the two strands. Transcription and DNA replication is inhibited if the two DNA strands are unable to separate completely, thus interrupting the ability to syn-thesize new protein required for cellular activity.

At high doses cyclophosphamide is cytotoxic to fast growing cells, whereas at low doses, CTX toxic activity is specific towards the elimination of inducer Helper T-cells. This will shift the ratio between helper/suppresser T-cells, causing a downregulation of the immune system. Although CTX is use frequently in autoimmune diseases, its use in graft rejection is limited due to the toxicities associated with its employment. Myelosuppression is an unacceptable adverse event, which may predispose the patient to oppor-tunistic infections.

METHOTREXATE

Similar to both azathioprine and cyclophosphamide, methotrexate (MTX) is also a chemotherapeutic agent that inhibits the biosynthesis of DNA, preventing clonogenic expansion. The mechanism by which methotrexate exerts its biological activity is different from azathioprine or cyclophosphamide. It does not exert its activity directly on the DNA synthesis; rather it is a dihydrofolate reductase (DHFR) competitive antagonist. DHFR is required to con-vert oxidized folate (dihydrofolate) to tetrahydrofolate. The inhibition of DHFR can inhibit nucleotide synthesis because tetrahydrofolate acid is a methylating agent that converts uridine to thymidine. A blockade of thymidine synthesis will reduce DNA synthesis causing cellular tox-icity in rapidly replicating cells. At doses of 10–25 mg/m², MTX is able to provide synergistic activity in combination with immunophilin binding and/or corticosteroid.

Immunophilin Binding Agents

Immunophilin binding agents (IBAs) are a group of agents that structurally heterogeneous, yet are biologically similar in that they bind to cytosolic receptors. These agents are immunosuppressive without cytotoxic or cytolytic activity. Rather IBAs suppress immune activation by selectively altering immunoregulatory activity.

All IBAs bind onto these intracellular receptors which have peptide-prolyl-cis-trans isomerase (PPIase) activity. The binding of IBAs onto the the cytosolic receptors, called immunophilins, inhibits the transduction signal required to activate transcription of cytokines important for lymphocyte activation and expansion. IBAs binding onto intracellular cytosolic receptors inhibit the isomerization of proline on peptidyl-proline bonds, causing improper protein folding that can terminate transduction signals. The ultimate re-sult of this is termination of transcription of lymphokines, thus suppressing lymphocyte proliferation.

CYCLOSPORINE

Cyclosporine belongs to a family of cyclic undecapeptides derived from a soil fungus (*Tolypolectin inflatum*). Because it is a cyclic peptide, it is a hydrophobic agent that is soluble in oils such as olive oil and cremaphor. This was the first IBA isolated and was found to have specific immuno-suppressive activity without killing the target lymphocytes. Cyclosporine A (CSA) exerts its immunosuppressive action by inhibiting the transcription of immunostimulating cyto-kines such as IL-2, IL-3, IL-5, IL-6, and GM-CSF. Although it is able to inhibit a myriad of cytokines, its ability to inhibit transcription of IL-2 seems to be the most impor-tant pharmacological activity.

CSA primarily targets CD4 lymphocytes, which are regu-lators of immunoactivation. It prevents mitogenic trans-duction signals after antigen binding onto the TCR. The resultant effect is decreased mRNA synthesis for transcription of IL-2 and other cytokines. In addition, CSA is able to inhibit transcription of IL-2 receptors (IL-2R) which reduce the sensitivity to IL-2 that is found in the circulation.

Biochemically, CSA inhibits transduction signals originating from the cellular membrane to the nucleus. This is accomplished through the binding of CSA onto intracellular receptors called cyclosporin binding protein or cyclophilin. Cyclophilin possesses enzymatic activity, and is called peptide-prolyl cis-trans isomerase (PPIase). This enzyme catalyzes protein folding and inhibition of the enzyme can lead to disruption of the transduction signal that is required for transcription activation and ultimately immunoactivation. Lymphocyte activation is dependent on both cytokine secretion and immune amplification. CSA interrupts the signals that prompts the synthesis of cytokines required for T-cell expansion.

Other biochemical activities of CSA include modifying genes that are important in multiple drug resistance (MDR) against chemotherapeutic agents. MDR is a P-glycoprotein that is responsible for reducing drug accumulation by actively pumping out cytotoxic drugs, such that intracellular levels are inadequate for cytotoxicity. P-glycoprotein is thought to be a calcium dependent pump which is inhibited by CSA's ability to block calcium release.

TACROLIMUS (FK506)

Tacrolimus or FK506, a member of the macrolide family, is structurally similar to erythromycin. This lactone macrolide is also an IBA similar to CSA. It differs from CSA in that it has its own intracellular receptor that is similar to cyclophilin, which is called FK506 binding protein or FKBP. Similiar to cyclophilin, FKBP has PPIase activity, which may explain why these two agents have similar activity yet are structurally different. FK506 binding of FKBP inhibits the isomerization of proline. This may be a rate-limiting step required for complex proteins to attain their fully active form. *In vitro*, FK506 is 100 times more immunosuppressive than CSA.

RAPAMYCIN

Rapamycin (RPM) is structually similar to FK506; however RPM consists of a 31-membered macrocyclic lactone whereas FK506 is a 23-membered macrocyclic lactone. RPM is another macrolide with immunosuppressive activity 1000 times more potent than CSA. RPM is similar to other IBAs, where immunosuppression does not require cytolytic activity. Unlike other immunosuppressants, RPM suppresses not only immune cells but also selective non-immune cells, such as smooth muscle and endothelial cells.

The structural difference between FK506 and RPM may explain why RPM is able to interfere with complex cytoplasmic biochemical cascades that transduce signals further down the intracellular signal pathway. This is evidenced by the fact that RPM remains active despite resistance towards FK506 and CSA, which may be due to RPM's ability to suppress thymocyte proliferation and B-cell activation as well.

Mycophenolic Acid

Mycophenolic acid (MPA) is a fermentation by-product of *Penicillin sp.* MPA inhibits inosine monophosphate dehydrogenase (IMPDH), an enzyme that catalyzes *de nova* synthesis of purine. Unlike other purine synthesis inhibitors, MPA is not a nucleoside, and does not require phosphorylation for activity. Furthermore, MPA does not inhibit DNA repair nor produce chromosomal breakage like purine analogs. Rather, MPA is a non-competitive reversible inhibitor of IMPDH that has the capacity to inhibit humoral and cellular immunity, by inhibiting T- and B-cell proliferation. Its ability to inhibit B-lymphocytes may explain why there is a reduction of serum antibodies.

Antibody Therapy

Antibody therapy is used to eliminate the cells responsible for cytotoxic activity or immunoactivation. Presently there are three types of antibodies that are approved for clinical use, OKT3, Antithymocyte globulin or antilymphocyte globulin (ATG/ALG), and Xomazyme H65 all of which work by eliminating CD3 cells. OKT3 and Xomozyme H65 are both monoclonal antibodies directed against CD3. The major difference between the OKT3 and Xomazyme H65 is that Xomazyme H65 is a monoclonal antibody conjugated with ricin-A. Unlike Xomazyme H65, OKT3 is a murine monoclonal antibody that is directed against the CD3, which utilizes the reticular endothelial system to eliminate opsonized circulating CD3 cells.

OKT3

OKT3 is a murine monoclonal antibody that is directed against CD3 surface antigen found on both CD4 and CD8 lymphocytes. Following administration of the OKT3, there is a rapid depletion of circulating T-lymphocytes, where the antibody binding will initiate cellular clearance when the opsonized cells pass through the reticular endothelial system. However the rapid clearance of circulating T-cells may cause overimmunosuppression which increases risk of developing opportunistic infections. Other problems associated with OKT3 include serum sickness because it is derived from murine source.

XOMAZYME H65

Xomazyme H65 (H65) is also a murine derived monoclonal antibody that is directed against CD3. Unlike OKT3, H65 is an immunotoxin, where the CD3 antibody is conjugated with ricin-A, a toxin that is derived from castor beans. The intact ricin molecule consists of an A- and B-subunit, where the A-subunit mediates the cellular toxicity. The B-subunit is the anchoring portion of the toxin allowing the A-subunit to elicit its cytotoxic effects. The monoclonal antibody substitutes for the B-subunit, thus producing a selective toxin.

ANTITHYMOCYTE GLOBULIN

Antilymphocyte globulin (ALG) is a polyclonal antibody that is derived from immunizing animals such as horses and sheep, with human lymphocytes. When thymocytes are used to immunize animals, the polyclonal antibodies are referred to as antithymocyte globulin (ATG). When lymphocytes are used, the polyclonal antibodies are called antilymphocyte globulin (ALG). These antibodies primarily impair cell-mediated responses by eliminating cellular binding. The reduction of lymphocytes is thought to be the primary action of ALG and ATG; however, the exact mechanism of action is still not fully understood.

The major problem associated with ALG/ATG therapy is that the preparations are not standardized, thus immunosuppressive activity varies from preparation to preparation. The optimal dose for immunosuppressive activity is therefore unknown. Another problem associated with ALG therapy is that the polyclonal antibodies are not selective for T-lymphocytes, thus crossreactivity to other hematological cells leading to thrombocytopenia may also occur. Furthermore, these antibodies are derived from animals, so crossreactions between animals and humans may result in a humoral response leading to serum sickness.

Cytokine Inhibitor Therapy

During graft rejection process, there is an elevation of pro-inflammatory cytokines like IL-1 and TNF. This is often accompanied by increased levels of interleukin-6 (IL-6), which can be induced by the presence of high levels of IL-1. The high levels of inflammatory mediators may activate prostaglandin synthesis which can explain some of the clinical signs and symptoms, such as fever, chills and rigors. High levels of prostaglandins and tissue damage may explain pain at the transplanted site.

Cytokines may also mobilize leukocytes from the walls of the vasculature and bone marrow. Cellular mobilization is accompanied by the clonal expansion stimulated by the presence of cytokines. In addition, cytokines will provide the chemotactic signals to enhance chemotaxis to the transplanted allograft.

At the site of graft rejection, there is infiltration of lymphocytes, which are predominately CTLs and NK cells. These cells are activated by the presence of IL-2, IL-12, and IFN-γ. However, the induction of all these cytokines is induced by the presence of IL-1 and TNF. Thus the blockade of the initial cytokine stimulus may inhibit the cytokine storm that will result in cellular attack of the allograft.

INTERLEUKIN-1 RECEPTOR ANTAGONIST

Interleukin-1 receptor antagonist (IL-1ra) is a naturally occurring cytokine that is structurally similar to both IL-1α and β. IL-1ra is 30% structurally homologous with IL-1; it differs from both IL-1 α and β in that it does not induce any pro-inflammatory activity. It is a competitive antagonist of both IL-1 α and IL-1 β. IL-1ra will bind onto IL-1 receptor (IL-1R) without inducing the intracellular signals required for lymphokine production. The exact mechanism by which IL-1ra exerts its activity is still uncertain; however, IL-1ra is able to block IL-1 induced expression of IL-6 and other cytokines as well.

The ability to block pro-inflammatory activity may be ameliorated if not prevented the graft rejection process. The inhibition of IL-1-like activity may also inhibit the expresssion of TNF, which is the other inflammatory mediator. Without cytokine activation, antigen binding onto TCR will not produce an intracellular signal that is adequate for immune activation.

The use of IL-1ra is not limited to graft rejection. It has been investigated in the treatment of various diseases that have elevated levels of IL-1. This includes autoimmune diseases such as rheumatoid arthritis, systemic lupus erythromatosus, irritable bowel syndrome, and myocarditis. Other areas where IL-1ra have been investigated include septic shock, AIDS-Kaposi's sarcoma, and acute myelogous leukemia. In all of these diseases, there is elevation of IL-1 where blockade of the IL-1 will block the autocrinic stimulus.

IL-1ra has been successfully used in the treatment of septic shock, and may eventually receive clinical approval for the treatment of this disease. In AIDS-KS and AML, patients have high levels of IL-1 which induce the expression of cytokines that provide the mitogenic stimulus for uncontrolled proliferation. In the laboratory setting, IL-1ra was able to block proliferation of AIDS-KS and AML.

ANTI-INTERLEUKIN-1 AND ANTI-TUMOR NECROSIS FACTOR

Pro-inflammatory cytokines such as IL-1 and TNF are elevated during the rejection process. A reduction of these cytokines has been shown to ameliorate the rejection process. Thus antibodies have been produced to eliminate immunoactivating cytokines, like IL-1 and TNF. The strategy here is to reduce the cytokine stimulus that is required for immunoactivation. Despite antigen binding onto TCR, the elimination of co-stimulation with cytokine activation results in anergy or no immune response.

SOLUBLE TUMOR NECROSIS FACTOR RECEPTORS

The body produces various soluble factors, which will mediate the downregulating of the immune system. As mentioned above, IL-1ra competitively binds IL-1R without activating pro-inflammatory activity. Although no naturally occurring receptor antagonist has been isolated for TNF, non-membrane bound TNF receptors have been found in the circulation, called soluble TNF receptors (STNFR). Presently, there are various types of STNFR, which may be called P55 and P75 because they are proteins with molecular weight of 55 and 75 kDs, respectively.

The soluble receptors act like cytokine sponges and compete with cellular receptors. Instead of competing for the receptors like IL-1ra, these soluble receptors compete for cytokines, thus reducing the signals for pro-inflammatory activation.

INTERLEUKIN-10

Unlike both IL-1ra and STNFR, interleukin-10 (IL-10) is not a competitive inhibitor. IL-10 exerts its biological activity by stimulating transduction that inhibits the synthesis of immunoactivating cytokines. Moreover, IL-10 is also able to stimulate the expression of IL-1ra, which will facilitate synergistic blockade of immune activation. In animals, IL-10 was able to block LPS mediated septic shock where the administration of LPS is able to activate both IL-1 and TNF. The precise mechanism of how IL-10 is able to mediate its activity is still unclear. More study is required to ascertain the biological activity of IL-10 in transplantation rejection. ■

References

- **Berke G.** (1997). Killing mechanisms of cytotoxic lymphocytes. *Curr Opin Hematol*, **4**(1), 32–40
- **Garivoy MR, Stock P, Bumgardner G, Keith F, Linker C.** (1994). Clinical Transplantation. In *Basic and Clinical Immunology Eight Edition*, edited by DP Stites, AI Terr, TG Parslow. Norwalk, Connecticut: Appleton & Lange, pp. 744–763
- **Halloran PF.** (1997). Immunosuppressive agents in clinical trials in transplantation. *Am. J. Med. Sci.*, **313**(5), 283–8
- **Knechtle SJ, Zhai Y, Fechner J.** (1996). Gene therapy in transplantation. *Transpl. Immunol.*, **4**(4), 257–64
- **Kohn DB.** (1996). Gene therapy for hematopoietic and immune disorders. *Bone Marrow Transplant.*, **18** Suppl 3, S55–8
- **Lui SL, Halloran PF.** (1996). Mycophenolate mofetil in kidney transplantation. *Current Opinion In Nephrology And Hypertension*, **5**(6), 5
- **Nash RA, Storb R.** (1996). Graft-versus-host effect after allogeneic hematopoietic stem cell transplantation: GVHD and GVL. *Curr. Opin. Immunol.*, **8**(5), 674–80
- **Orosz CG.** (1996). Networked alloimmunity: a brief reexamination of some basic concepts in transplantation immunobiology. *J. Heart. Lung. Transplant.*, **15**(11), 1063–8
- **Platt JL.** (1996). Xenotransplantation: recent progress and current perspectives. *Curr. Opin. Immunol.*, **8**(5), 721–8
- **Shapiro R.** (1997). Tacrolimus (FK-506) in kidney transplantation. *Transplant. Proc.*, **29**(1–2), 45–7
- **Tutschka P, Santos G,** *et al.* (1980). *Immunobiology of Bone Marrow Transplantation*. New York: Springer Verlag, pp. 375.
- **Winkelstine A.** (1994). Immunosuppressive Therapy. In *Basic and Clinical Immunology Eight Edition*, edited by DP Stites, AI Terr, TG Parslow. Norwalk, Connecticut: Appleton & Lange, pp. 765–780

Case Study with Self-Assessment Question

JC is a 48 year old male who has been on business in a small country in Africa for the last three months. While in Africa, a malaria epidemic began spreading throughout the small country. The American embassy recommended that all travelers within the country take chloroquine (Anti-malarial agent) for prevention against malaria. JC was well throughout his stay in Africa, and continued on chloroquine prophylaxis for an additional week after his return. Upon return, JC complained of chills and fever, and took some chloramphenicol that he had obtained overseas. His fevers persisted for another 5 days. He entered into the emergency room and was assessed for possible pneumonia. On physical examination, JC was found to have severe bruising on his back. He denies any trauma to that area, but claimed that he was on his back for the last 3 days. Additionally, he was found to have gum bleeding. His laboratory values were notable for pancytopenia. A bone marrow was performed and the initial report suggested that the patient may have chloroquine or chloramphenicol-induced acute leukemia.

Chest X-ray: Patchy infiltrate with consolidation in the left lower lobe, consistent with possible aspiration pneumonia.

Chest: Rales and ronchi.

Vital signs: Bp: 85/45   HR: 132   Tmax 39.2°C   RR   32

Physical Exam: Hacking cough with productive sputum.

Throat: Tender to touch with enlarged lymph nodes.

Allergies: Sulfur drugs and penicillin (Rash)

Laboratory:

Na	135(135–145)	Cl	108(101–111)	BUN	89 (7–22)	Glu	120 (70–110)
K	4.2 (3.5–5.0)	CO_2	20.4 (24–32)	Scr	3.1 (0.7–1.3)		
Ca	9.2 (8.2–10.6)	PO_4	3.2 (2.5–4.5)	Mg	2.1 (1.7–2.5)		
TPro	7.1 (6.0–8.0)	Alb	4.2 (3.2–5.5)	Tbili	0.7 (0.0–1.3)		
AP	119 (20–100)	AST	450 (5–40)	ALT	323 (5–40)		
LDH	82 (100–250)	UA	4.5 (3.5–7.2)				
WBC	1.3 (4.1–10.9)	Hgb	8.3 (13–16)	Hct 25.1 (40–50)			

Sputum gram stain: Few epithelial, 3+ gram negative bacilli, and 1+ gram positive cocci. White blood cells: many.

Sputum culture: Pending.

Blood culture: Gram negative bacilli, suspected Pseudomonas sp. Final report to follow.

Question 1:   *The patient later develops acute leukemia, which requires that he receive an allogeneic BMT. His pre-existing marrow was abrogated with a combination of cyclophosphamide, busulfan, and etoposide. He is now day 1 status post-allogenenic BMT from his HLA-matched brother. His physicians recommended an immunosuppressive regimen of cyclosporine A 2 mg/kg/day IVPB continuous, methylprednisolone 80 mg IVP qd, and methotrexate 30 mg qd IV or PO. Is this regimen adequate for immunosuppressive therapy to prevent graft versus host disease?*

Answer 1:   This regimen is for patients who are receiving an allogenic bone marrow transplant. The combination of cyclosporine and prednisone is the back-bone to this immunosuppressive regimen. Cyclosporine inhibits the expression and secretion of interleukin-2 (IL-2), which is the immune activator of graft rejection. Prednisone is a glucocorticoid, which inhibits the proliferation of lymphocytes that include cytotoxic T-lymphocytes. Thus the two drugs reduce the number of cells that are responsible for graft rejection, and cytokine stimuli that activates the immune system. Because this patient is over 35 years of age, the addition of methotrexate is necessary. This is because patients who are over 35 years old have a greater propensity for developing graft versus host disease. The doses that are employed are within the recommended dosage; however, cyclosporine levels are necessary to ensure that they are within the therapeutic range.

9 Vaccines

Introduction

In ancient history, it was found that individuals who survived a disease seldom suffered from a secondary exposure towards that same disorder. This protective effect led to deliberate inoculation where smallpox scabs were first used as a vaccine more than three centuries ago in China and India. However, the birth of vaccine immunology as a science may be dated back to Edward Jenner's successful vaccination against smallpox reported in 1798. Jenner noted that milkmaids who had pockmarks on their hands, consistent with cowpox, did not develop smallpox. He proceeded to study the protective effect of cowpox by deliberately inoculating an 8 year old boy, who was later exposed to smallpox. The boy failed to develop smallpox despite repeated inoculation with pus from smallpox lesions.

The importance of prophylactic immunization against infectious diseases is best illustrated by the fact that worldwide programs of vaccination have led to the complete or near complete eradication of many of these diseases in developed countries. Smallpox is perhaps the most impressive example where the incidence is near totally eradicated. The development of effective vaccines against virus, bacteria, and parasite remains an important global objective. The aim of all vaccination is to induce specific immunity that prevents microbial invasion, eliminates microbial entrance into the host, and neutralizes microbial toxins that are present in the circulation.

Immune Response Primary Exposure

Immune response to primary antigenic exposure requires processing and presentation of the antigen to helper T-lymphocytes. Processing of the antigen requires precious time that may allow the pathogen to proliferate. When the immune system has adequately responded to the foreign intrusion, clinical manifestations may have already induced significant tissue damage.

While primary immune response is normally slow, secondary exposure to the same antigen is much more rapid than the initial exposure. This is attributed to the presence of memory lymphocytes, which bypass the lengthy antigen processing and presentation processes. Sensitized individuals respond more rapidly and with greater intensity to prevent the onset of clinical disease.

Humoral response to primary antigen challenge differs from secondary exposure. In primary exposure, IgM antibodies are predominate with IgG rising days after initial humoral response. A delay in IgG elevation is attributed to the time required for antigen processing, which may explain why IgG are more specific than IgM. In primary exposure, blood concentrations of IgM and IgG are comparable during the initial antigenic exposure. However, during secondary exposure the IgG response is faster and more intensive when compared to the primary immune response. During secondary exposure, the concentration of IgG response can be 2–10 times higher than primary exposure (Figure 9.1).

Cellular Response During Secondary Antigenic Exposure

Typically, the primary immune response is rapidly downregulated after the elimination of the antigen. However, in situations such as infections, sustained immune response can occur especially when microorganisms are difficult to eradicate. In most circumstances, the majority of effector cells that are generated are quickly eliminated from the circulation. Similarly, the majority of the circulating B-lymphocytes are cleared within 1–2 weeks.

The rapid removal of effector cells may have a beneficial effect, where redundant cells are removed. Maintaining high levels of redundant cells can cause excessive tissue injury when a second exposure occurs. In addition, progressive accumulation of effector cells can overload host capacity, such that the immune response may be delayed.

Removal of redundant cells is unquestioned; however, the elimination process must be selective such that important elements are maintained to respond effectively in the event of re-exposure. After eliminating a majority of the circulating lymphocytic clones, a sub-population of both T- and B-lymphocytes will persist. These persistent cells are referred to as "memory cells," which provide the means

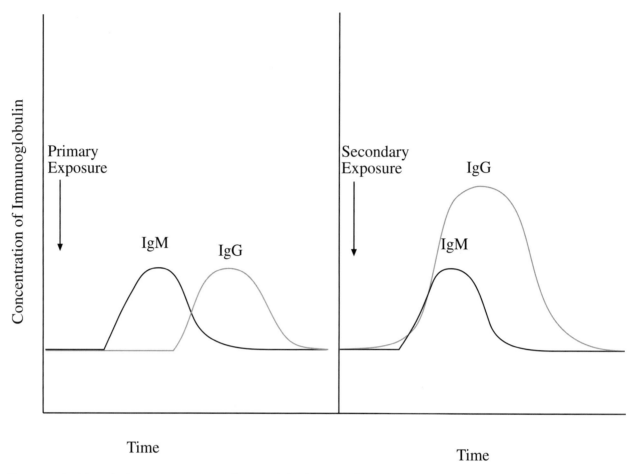

Figure 9.1. Initial antibody response is primarily IgM, while elevation of IgG concentration occurs later. The antibody response is altered in a secondary exposure to the same antigen. In this scenario, the concentration of IgG is 2–10 times higher than primary exposure. In addition, the IgG response occurs with a much smaller lag time as compared to the primary antigenic exposure. These changes may be attributed to the presence of memory lymphocytes following initial exposure.

to bypass the antigen processing and presentation in the event of re-exposure.

There is some controversy as to the nature of antigenic affinity of these cells, where low affinity cells are referred to as immature cells, and high antigenic affinity suggests more mature clones. For T-lymphocytes, the memory CTLs have high affinity for cells bearing the antigen. Long-lived memory B-lymphocytes also seem to be mature lymphocytes with high affinity for the antigen. Thus persistent cells are not only responsive, but are highly antigenic specific.

Duration of Immunity

Exposure to certain microorganisms can provide lifelong immunity against these pathogens; however, the immunological duration of response may differ and are dependent on the types of organism. Certain exposures can confer lifelong immunity where a signal exposure will produce a durable response, such as measles, mumps and chickenpox. Other types of microorganisms such as tuberculosis and tetanus may only provide protection over a short period and thereby required repeat immunization.

The duration of immunity is dependent on the different subtypes of T- and B-lymphocytes that are sensitized. This may be in response to the various types cells that are formed during initial antigenic priming. Several variables may influence the duration of immunity, including the concentration of the antigen, the number of exposures, and the duration of immune priming. Dose and route of exposure may also play a role in the duration of immunity. All of these factors are important in the priming and the selection of specific clones. The properties of the antigen may, itself, play an important role in eliciting immune response.

Vaccines

Newborns have little immunity against pathogens found in the environment. Other than maternal immunoglobulins, newborns have no immune defense mechanism and are at the mercy of infectious organisms present in the environment. Passive immunity could be conferred by the oral administration of maternal milk containing protective immunoglobulins. However, active immunity can only be conferred by direct antigenic exposure that will initiate immune priming, thus producing memory against the pathogen. When an infectious organism is administered to an individual, this can be considered as a deliberate active immunization or vaccination.

Following Jenner's initial findings, little was done to further describe the protective nature of deliberate immunization. Not until Louis Pasteur's discovery that sheep inoculated with heat treated anthrax bacilli could confer protection against virulent bacilli was there any advancement in vaccine technology. The heating process was able to weaken or attenuate the anthrax such that the immunological response was conferred without developing full-blown clinical disease. The weakened anthrax was immunogenic enough to prime the immune system, yet unable to produce physiological signs of infection. This discovery suggested that clinical disease was not necessary for immune priming. Instead, antigen exposure was all that was necessary to prime the immune system.

Vaccination has the capacity to protect the immunized patient by priming the immunological defense against a secondary exposure. Vaccines are immunogens capable of stimulating the host immune system, where deliberate exposure to the antigen results in the production of memory B- and T-lymphocytes against the specific target. A patient is adequately immunized when a second exposure enables the individual to more rapidly respond to the antigen with both humoral and cellular components. This accelerated immune response enables the host to neutralize the pathogen before the infectious burden can produce significant cellular injury. Thus, the purpose of a vaccine is to either prevent or reduce acute clinical manifestation of infection.

Types of Vaccines

Various types of vaccines exists, and are classified as either live or inactivated vaccines (Table 9.1). Live vaccines are organisms that replicate in the immunized patient, but are less pathogenic because they have been attenuated. Inactivated vaccine may be either killed organisms or purified fractions of a representative pathogen.

There are both advantages and disadvantages associated with either type of vaccine. Live attenuated vaccines

Live vaccines	Inactivated vaccines
1. Live attenuated	1. Chemically inactivated
• Chemical	2. Heat inactivated
• Heat	3. Irradiation inactivated
• Irradiated	4. Isolated secreted proteins
2. Non-pathogenic mutant	5. Anti-idiotype antibodies
3. Related non-pathogenic species	6. Cellular fractionation
4. Recombinant live vaccines	

Table 9.1. Various types of vaccines.

contain organisms that are less virulent than the organisms associated with disease, and may produce a subclinical infection. These vaccines are usually produced by attenuating a pathogen using either heat, irradiation, chemicals or a combination of agents. The attenuated organism is able to proliferate and thus provide a continual supply of antigen for priming. These organisms are able to proliferate and replicate; therefore they also have the capacity of reacquiring their virulence factor and causing disease. A major disadvantage of live attenuated vaccine is the potential to revert back to a pathogenic state.

Less virulent organisms may also exist in nature, thus isolation of low virulence mutants has also been used as a means to produce vaccines. The first reported vaccine by Edward Jenner used a related virus to inoculate patients against smallpox, where cowpox did not have significant morbidity associated with human exposure. Similarly, the use of a related non-pathogenic microorganism may be a good candidate for a live vaccine.

Inactivated vaccines are either organisms that are treated with high-energy irradiation, chemicals, heat, or a combination. The inactivated organism can be given intact or in a fractionated form. Inactivated vaccines can be produced by isolating the immunogenic fractions. These cellular fractions are usually antigens located on the surface of the pathogens. However, immunogenic fractions can also be secreted products such as toxins or enzymes. The major advantage of cellular subunit vaccines is that they are incapable of reacquiring virulence factor, because they are not intact cells. Conversely, this decreases their ability to provide a continuous supply of antigens for immunological priming.

1.	Able to mimic the immunological response as if an actual pathogenic incursion.
2.	Induce immune response as true infections.
3.	Able to provide a continuous supply of antigen
4.	Immunological activation of both cellular and humoral response • B-lymphocytes expansion • T-lymphocytes expansion. • Elevation of antigen specific IgG. • Durable life-long memory

Table 9.2. Characteristics of an ideal vaccine.

Characteristics of an Ideal Vaccine

There are several characteristics that define an ideal vaccine. An ideal vaccine is one that is able to mimic the immunological response as if it was an actual pathogenic incursion (Table 9.2). Immunological activation should include both a cellular and humoral response, where there are signs of B- and T-lymphocytes expansion. An elevation of antigen specific IgG is essential, indicating that there has been T-cell priming and activation. The immunological response elicited by the vaccine should be durable such that daily or even monthly administration is unnecessary. Ideally, vaccine immunization should provide life-long protection. Other important features of an ideal vaccine are that the immunogenic effect should not be offset by side effects such as a clinical manifestation. The ability to produce a continuous and low dose antigenic challenge should provide a sustained and durable immunological response, thus circumventing clinical disease. An Ideal vaccine should also lack any long-term undesirable effects such as reactivation and the activation of cancer development. Thus the ability to reacquire virulence should be eliminated completely to prevent such an incidence from occurring.

Attenuated Live – Vaccines

Live attenuated vaccines were the first agents described to confer specific immunity. The goal of attenuated vaccines is to prime the immune system to respond against the desired organism without the development of disease. These vaccines consist of weakened or attenuated organisms that can proliferate and provide a continuous antigen to the host. Patients who receive attenuated vaccine may develop sub-clinical disease where symptoms are less intensive compared actual infections.

The earliest described immunization was achieved by scratching a small amount of dried and pulverized small-pox scabs. Scratching the skin of the patient with this mixture is similar to intradermal inoculation. The majority of the inoculated patients developed mild signs of clinical diseases, while a few individuals actually developed full-blown disease. Although an attenuated organism is normally less viable and replicates at a slower rate, such organisms have the potential to regain their virulence and precipitate acute signs and symptoms of infection. This may explain why some patients developed full-blown disease.

There are several methods in the development of attenuate live vaccines. One is the isolation of either a non-virulent or less-virulent mutant. In nature, there are organisms that are either related species or from the same species, but are less virulent than the pathogenic strain. These mutants are ideal as vaccines because they are able to mimic the natural infection process without causing the same type of symptoms. These organisms are able to elicit a durable immune response, because they provide a continuous source of antigen.

Pathogens can be attenuated using heat, high energy waves, or chemicals to weaken their ability to produce clinical disease. Mutations can be induced by exposure to high energy waves, that causes damage to the DNA. Both gamma radiation (x-rays) and ultraviolet (uv) waves can attenuate the virulence; exposure to short pulses can induce mutant forms that are less virulent than the wild-type organism. Chemicals can also induce mutational changes similar to high energy waves.

After wild-type organisms are attenuated, selection of the best candidate is needed. The candidate vaccine should have a stable mutation that is unable to regain its virulence. However, the attenuated organism must be able to proliferate in the host to provide antigenic challenge, which will prime the immune system. Even though the attenuated organism is a stable mutant that can proliferate in the host, the antigens that it expresses must provide protection against the wild type organism. In order to ensure this, similar surface antigens must be present to provide the protective response.

Recently, biotechnology has been used to attenuate pathogens either by adding or "knocking out" a gene in these organisms. A gene can be added to the wild type organism that will inhibit its normal proliferation. Conversely, genes that are crucial for replication can either be selectively deleted or mutated to weaken the organism. After the organisms have been genetically altered, these candidate vaccines must be screened for ability to replicate in animals and ability to cause disease. Immune response to the attenuated organism can be measured by the presence of specific IgG directed against the wild type organism. Cellular response should also be demonstrated where the primed cells are able to exert a cytotoxic effect against the wild-type organism. This can be demonstrated by adding effector cells into radiolabeled wild-type organisms. Radiolabelling the cell free supernatant will allow measurement of cytotoxic activity.

Inactivated Vaccines

KILLED VACCINES

Unlike attenuated vaccines, inactivated vaccines contain non-replicating organisms or cellular fractions, thus the risk of direct vaccine induced disease is minimal. Without proliferation, these vaccines cannot provide the continuous antigenic challenge that is important for immunological priming. In addition, inactivated vaccines are usually less effective when compared to attenuated vaccines for the same antigen. Less immunogenicity may be the reason for inactivate vaccines being less effective. Decreased immunogenicity may be attributed to disruption of the natural conformation of the antigen. Other effects include antigen breakdown or interaction with other cellular elements. Although the potential for direct vaccine induced disease is minimal, it is impossible to ensure that all organisms are completely inactivated without destroying the antigen(s).

There are various techniques to inactivate or kill organisms. The major difference is the intensity and the duration of the treatment, these are similar to those used to attenuate microorganisms. Microorganisms can be heat-killed, or chemically disrupted such that the intact cells are completely destroyed. An alternative method is to treat the cells with irradiation, which maintains cellular structure but still kills the cells. High energy irradiation can cause DNA fragmentation leading to DNA endonuclease activation, and to total chromosomal breakdown. The nuclei of irradiated cells are filled with fragmented chromosomes; however, the immunogenic cellular structure may be intact.

Loss of cellular structure may reduce the amount of immunogens that are available for immune sensitization. Reduced immune exposures are another reason why inactivated vaccines are less active than live vaccines. Here vaccine adjuvants are added to improve their immunogenicity. Because adjuvants are usually made of aluminum compounds, they can also serve as emulsifying agents that may act as a drug delivery system. The emulsified vaccines are mixed with adjuvant, and release small amounts to the body, thus acting like a depot delivery system.

FRACTIONATED PROTEIN

Since vaccines are immunogens that are cellular components, it is understandable that only the immunogenic components are necessary. The cellular component can serve as a vaccine. This can be accomplished by isolating only the immunogenic fraction(s) of the pathogen. Disruption of the cellular structure using either mechanical, chemical, or high energy techniques is followed by isolation of the cellular fraction.

If the desired fraction is on the cellular surface, the disrupted cellular mixture is centrifuged in a density gradient. The membranes are then isolated after removal of the cystolic and nuclear fractions. Because the cellular membrane is a mosaic of glycoproteins, proteins, lipids and glycolipids, the cellular membrane fraction must be further fractionated. This can be accomplished using column chromatography (Figure 9.2). Chromatographic methods exploit the ionic, size, and hydrophilicity properties of the cellular subunits in order to separate them. The desired fractions are collected and are tested for their ability to prime the immune system.

There are other methods of producing cellular fractions that can be accomplished using recombinant techniques. After the cellular component(s) are isolated, the immunogenic fractions are digested into smaller fragments using degradation enzymes. The digested proteins are separated to isolate these peptide fragments. A selected number of peptides undergo sequence analysis. From the amino acid sequence, a degenerative nucleotide sequence consisting of approximately 30 nucleotides is synthesized. These nucleotide sequences can be used as complementary nucleotide probes in the genome containing that sequence. This is accomplished when the probe binds onto the complement regions within the genome.

The entire genome can be obtained using salt extraction. After total DNA or RNA is isolated, various genes can be separated using electrophoresis. This uses an electric field to move the nucleotide sequence through a gel matrix. The separated DNA/RNA is then transferred onto a nitrocellulose or nylon filter, and crosslinked using UV-irradiation.

Once the separated nucleotide sequence cross-links onto a filter, radioactive probes such as those mentioned above are added to a solution that will interact with the filter. The complement nucleotide sequence binds onto the filter. A DNA library is established and sequenced to identify the gene encoding for the desire protein. Genes that produce proteins with the same size and physical features are analyzed to ensure that the correct gene has been selected.

Once the gene has been isolated, it can be copied in large quantities using gene amplification techniques. The desire gene is then inserted into producer cells by joining the gene together with a gene vector, which is usually derived from bacterial plasmids or viral genomes. The recombinant vector is reinserted into an expression cell system. *E. Coli* and *Saccharomyces cerevisiae* are the most frequently used expression cell systems because the cost of maintaining these organisms is relatively inexpensive. The desired cellular subunit is harvested and purified to homogeneity.

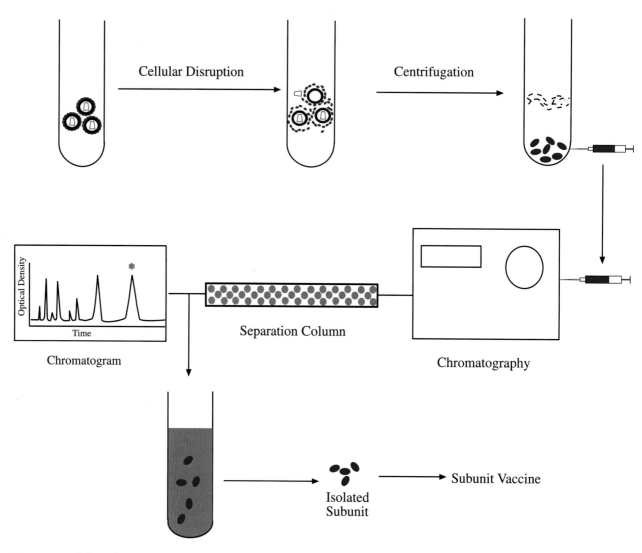

Figure 9.2. Cellular subunits can be isolated by disrupting the target organism with either solvent detergent or mechanical methods. The cell homogenate is then separated by centrifugation to isolated the membrane fraction. The membranes fractions are passed through a column chromatograph to further separate the immunogen.

The purified product is then tested for its ability to induce an immune response in animals. Following immunization, plasma is extracted to determine if IgG specific against the pathogen is produced. In addition, a cellular response is again assessed to determine if cell-mediated toxicity can be induced using the purified recombinant fraction. In the event of an immune response against the recombinant product not inducing sufficient immune priming, it can be formulated with adjuvants to enhance the immune response.

Anti-idiotype Vaccines

Vaccines have also been produced using antibody technology. Anti-idiotype antibodies have served as the immunogen.

As described in Chapter 2, anti-idiotype antibodies are secondary antibodies targeted against the antigen binding fragment or Fab of the primary antibody that is specific for a region on the antigen. Structurally, the private anti-idiotype antibody resembles the original antigen, and is utilized as the antigen to produce the vaccine (Figure 9.3).

Antiidiotype antibodies are produced by first immunizing animals with the primary antigen. Antigens inoculated into animals will direct its response against the immunogen. Spleens of immunized animals are removed to isolate antibody secreting B-lymphocytes or plasma cells. These cells are grown in culture and their supernatant analyzed for the presence of antibodies directed against the antigen.

Plasma cells have a limited life-span in culture despite subculturing the primary isolates. Thus immortalization of

Anti-idiotype
Antibody

Anti-idiotype
Antibody

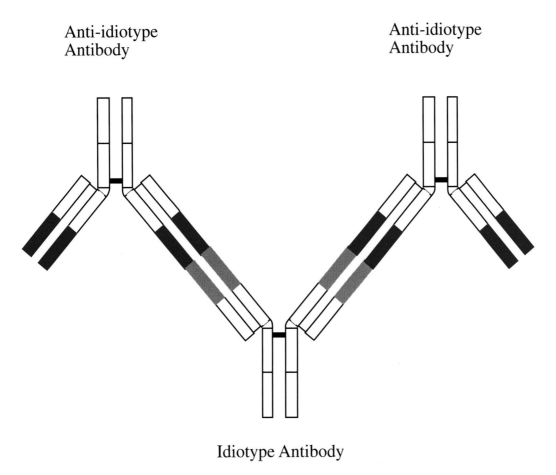

Idiotype Antibody

Figure 9.3. The various antigen binding sites of the same antigen is called the idiotype. Antibodies directed against the antigen binding site are referred to as anti-idiotype, where these antibodies are structurally similar to the original antigen, and thus can be utilized as a vaccine.

the isolated B-lymphocytes is necessary. Viral transformation or fusion with a myeloma cell can immortalize plasma cells. As mentioned in Chapter 2, when hybridoma technology is employed, the cellular mixture must be subcultured in HAT medium to isolate plasma/myeloma hybrids. The supernatant is analyzed for the presence of antibodies against the primary antigen.

When enough monoclonal antibodies directed against the antigen is produced, the antibodies are digested to form Fab and Fc components. The Fab is usually linked together as haptens to increase the immune response against the Fab, which is used to immunize a secondary animal. The plasma from the secondary animal is analyzed for the presence of immunoglobulin against the Fab fragments. The presence of anti-Fab will indicate the presence of anti-idiotype antibodies. The spleen of the secondary animal is removed and plasma cells are isolated and subcultured.

A number of plasma cells will bind onto the primary antibody's Fab, which are called anti-idiotype antibodies directed against the primary antibody. The structure of the

anti-idiotype can be structurally similar to the primary antigen, and thus are used as the immunogen against that pathogen. Once again, hybridoma technology is needed to mass produce enough product for clinical use.

Although this type of vaccine eliminates the chances of pathogen contamination, the cost of producing anti-idiotypes is expensive. Another limitation associated with both subunit and anti-idiotype vaccines is the high degree of specificity, which allows the targeted organism to evade the activated immune response by making small mutational changes.

Vaccinia Technology

Cowpox, being the first modern-day vaccine, is often referred to as vaccinia. Historically, vaccinia was used to immunize against smallpox. Immunity is conferred because cowpox is structurally similar to smallpox virus. Vaccinia is highly immunogenic, and is now also being used as a biological carrier for weakly immunogenic subunit particles. Utilizing DNA technology, genes are inserted into the vaccinia where the antigens are expressed on the surface of vaccinia carriers. Utilizing vaccinia as a carrier provides the advantage of attenuated vaccines where a continuous flow of antigens are challenging the immune system. Also, recombinant vaccinia can have more than one antigen used in a single carrier, where the insertion of a number of genes can result in the formation of a number of different immunological responses. Examples of where this type of technology is being used include investigational vaccines against respiratory syncytial virus, HIV, para-influenza, rotavirus, malaria, hepatitis B and herpes simplex virus.

HIV Vaccines

The development of vaccines against HIV is an important factor in stemming the spread of AIDS. There are several HIV vaccine candidates under development, which include live attenuated virus, subunits of HIV, anti-idiotype, and vaccinia virus.

An attenuated virus vaccine is an unlikely candidate for an HIV vaccine because of the nature of HIV infection. However, a killed-virus vaccine is currently under development. HIV infected patients with generalized lymphadenopathy were inoculated with γ-irradiated HIV immunogenic vaccine. An intradermal booster was given three months after the initial dose. Patients who were previously anergic became reactive towards the skin test, suggesting that killed-HIV immunization can restore the immune response.

An immunogenic subunit vaccine will circumvent the threat of inadvertent infection. Unlike attenuated or killed vaccines, these vaccines do not have intact organisms. Instead, the immunogenic subunits are produced using recombinant technology (Figure 9.4). The purified subunits are less immunogenic than whole virus vaccine, often requiring the addition of an adjuvant. Purified gp 120 has been shown to convey immunity. Chimpanzees immunized with gp 120 had effective antibody titers. With each subsequent dose, there was an elevation of antibody titer directed against gp120, suggesting that this agent may be a viable candidate vaccine.

Vaccines produced by vaccinia virus technology are undergoing clinical evaluation in patients with HIV. One such vaccinia expresses HIV envelope glycoprotein or *env-5*. Animals immunized with *env-5* vaccinia developed antibodies against *env* suggesting that *env-5*-vaccinia can induce specific immune response. More importantly, the emergence of HIV specific cytotoxic T-lymphocytes demonstrated that the cellular immune response can be stimulated. To assess the ability to protect against primary HIV infections, animals immunized with *env-5*-vaccinia were infected with HIV. No development of lymphadenopathy was apparent; however, viruses were isolated from both control and immunized groups. These results suggest that the immune system can control viral replication, but were unable to prevent primary infection.

Human studies using an *env*-vaccinia confirmed its ability to confer immunity by developing low levels of anti-HIV antibodies, and the presence of cellular immunity directed against HIV. Although antibodies were restricted to HIV-1, helper T-cell responsiveness had a broader activity against both HIV-1 and HIV-2. This evidence suggests that an impressive immune response can be produced in humans. In a follow-up study, the same volunteers previously immunized with *env*-vaccinia were given another recombinant vaccinia virus expressing fragments of gp120 (surface antigen on HIV), where 57% of the patients responded to the antigen challenge.

The expression of other HIV antigens on vaccinia carriers, such as expression of gp120 and gp160, is also able to induce immunity against HIV. Antibodies are reactive against HIV-1, and to a lesser extent HIV-2. The anti-gp 120 antibodies blocked virus attachment onto CD4, which is an important step in HIV infection.

Tumor Vaccine

There is compelling evidence demonstrating that activated immune system can control and/or eliminate tumor progression. Landmark studies using IL-2 showed tumors that were refractory to conventional therapy responded to IL-2 stimulation. The demonstration that immunoactivation can control tumor progression has spurred research into the development of tumor vaccines. Unlike other vaccines where the purpose is to prevent the onset or ameliorate clinical disease, the purpose of tumor vaccines is to prime the immune system to direct its attack on the tumor. The center of an effective tumor vaccine is the activation of cellular immunity, more specifically, the stimulation of cytotoxic T-lymphocyte activity.

A number of tumors are also linked to viral infections, where the inhibition of viral transformation can cause tumor to regress. Cellular immunity is important against both viral infections and tumor, thus the primary objective in tumor vaccines is to activate specific cellular immunity. Similar to other vaccines, tumor vaccines are usually derived from lysed primary tumor cells that can either be killed tumor tissue or fractionated subunits. Vaccine adjuvants are usually added to enhance immune priming. To improve the immune response, biological response modifiers to stimulate cellular response (such as IL-2 and IFN-α) are often used.

Although the majority of the tumor vaccines have been cellular fractions, the use of whole cells that are added into the patient's proliferating lymphocytes has been studied.

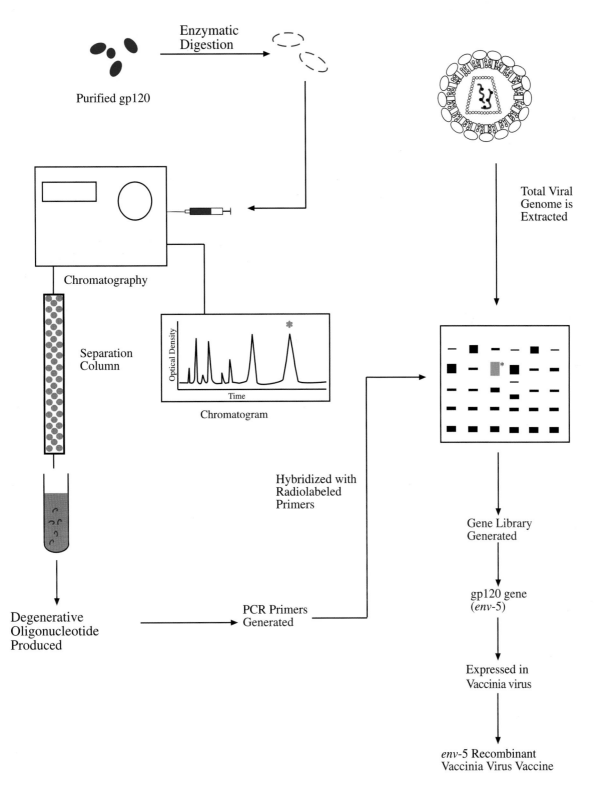

Figure 9.4. Purified gp120 was enzymatically digested into small peptide fragments. Digested gp120 was separated using column chromatography and the fragments were collected. Degenerative oligonucleotide primers were generated after protein sequencing. The primers are mass produced using polymerase chain reaction (PCR) techniques. Radiolabeled attached PCR products can be used as probes to isolate the viral gene encoding for gp120. A gene library is generated, and the entire gene is sequenced. The sequenced gene can be expressed in a virus such as vaccinia as carriers of the HIV surface antigen.

The entire lymphocyte population and tumor cells are infused back into the patient in hope of further priming the immune system to target on cells (tumor cells) with these antigens.

Vaccine Adjuvant

Immunogenic subunit vaccines circumvent the threat of inadvertent infection. Unlike killed vaccines, these vaccines are not intact organisms and unable to proliferate in the host, and thus unable to produce a continuous supply of antigen. Conversely, the administration of large doses of immunogens can cause potential intolerable immune effects. In these circumstances, the addition of chemicals that will enhance immunoactivation is employed. These agents are more commonly referred to as vaccine adjuvants, usually aluminum compounds, muramyl dipeptide, and Corynebacterium parvum.

Freund's complete adjuvant (FCA) is a suspension of mycobacteria in oil and detergent that stimulates the immune response towards weak immunogens. The mycobacterial oils act like a lipopolysaccharide by inducing macrophage activation. Detergents are used to disrupt the oils and keep the antigens and oils in suspension, resulting in slow release (Depot effect) of the antigen into the circulation. Although FCA is effective in stimulating the immune system, its effective is so intense that it is not recommended for human use.

Less intense adjuvants have been developed like muramyl dipeptide, and *Corynebacterium parvum* extract. These two products are similar to FCA in that they are bacterial extracts used to enhance the immune system. Like FCA, muramyl dipeptide is derived from mycobacterium, but is less immunoactivating. There are drawbacks associated with dose escalation of vaccine adjuvant, where overstimulated macrophages can increase the risk of lymphoid hyperplasia (Table 9.3).

Alums are the main vaccine adjuvants used clinically. Alums are aluminum containing compounds that enhance immunostimulation and also serve as antigen delivery systems, where antigens are slowly released. The major problem associated with alums has been pain at the site of injection. Other adjuvants include the used of biological response modifying agents such as interferons and interleukins. These biological adjuvants can specifically stimulate cellular immunity, where natural killer cells and cytotoxic T-lymphocytes are expanded and activated. ■

References

- **Ellis RW.** (1988). New technologies for making vaccines. In *Vaccines*, edited by SA Plotkin, EA Mortimer. Philadephia: W.B. Saunders Company, PA, pp. 568–575
- **Itoh K, Hayashi A, Toh Y, Imai Y, Yamada A, Nishida T, Shichijo S.** (1997). Development of cancer vaccine by tumor rejection antigens. *Int. Rev. Immunol.,* (2–3), 153–71
- **Morein B, Lovgren-Bengtsson K, Villacres-Eriksson M.** (1996). What to expect of future vaccines? *Acta. Vet. Scand. Suppl.,* **9**, 101–6
- **Robbins PF, Kawakami Y.** (1996). Human tumor antigens recognized by T cells. *Curr. Opin. Immunol.,* **8**(5), 628–36
- **Roy P.** (1996). Genetically engineered particulate virus-like structures and their use as vaccine delivery systems. *Intervirology,* **39**(1–2), 62–71
- **Russo S, Turin L, Zanella A, Ponti W, Poli G.** (1997). What's going on in vaccine technology? *Med. Res. Rev.,* **17**(3), 277–301
- **Shearer GM, Clerici M.** (1997). Vaccine strategies: selective elicitation of cellular or humoral immunity? *Trends Biotechnol.,* **15**(3), 106–9
- **Slifka MK, Ahmed R.** (1996). Long-term humoral immunity against viruses, revisiting the issue of plasma cell longevity. *Trends Microbiol.,* **4**(10), 394–400
- **Zhao Z, Leong KW.** (1996). Controlled delivery of antigens and adjuvants in vaccine development. *J. Pharm. Sci.,* **85**, 1261–70

Self-Assessment Questions

Question 1: *JJ is a 6 month old baby who comes into the clinic for his scheduled vaccination. He receives his second mumps, pertussis, and measles vaccine without incidence. Compare the immunological response in patients infected with measles who were vaccinated with mumps, measles, and pertussis as compared to those who were not vaccinated. Discuss and compare similarities and differences in terms of IgM and IgG response (You should consider the timing and intensity of Ig responses).*

Question 2: *Therapeutic VAX has developed a new tumor vaccine that the company claims will enable cancer patients to combat any type of malignant growth. You are a Food and Drug Administration inspector who is in charge of investigating this claim.*

You are told in Therapeutic VAXs report that Maxi VAX is a glycoprotein that was purified from the membranes of multiple myeloma cells (B-lymphocyte tumor). The company claims that the glycoprotein is found in all cells in the body, but is expressed in high quantities in malignant cells. What is your first impression of Therapeutic VAXs claims that it will be effective against all tumor types?

Answer 1: If JJ was infected with either mumps, measles, or pertussis prior to vaccination, his IgM would response first. The IgG response would be delayed as compared to the IgM response. The intensity of the IgM and IgG response in an unvaccinated individual is about the same.

However, if JJ was vaccinated with mumps, measles, and pertussis prior to being exposed, the IgM response would be similar as if he was never exposed. The difference would be an early response in IgG. The intensity of IgG response will be 2–10 fold higher than in a person who was not previously vaccinated.

Answer 2: If MaxiVAX is found in all cells, it would be highly unlikely that the body will produce an immunological response to this surface glycoprotein. This is because the body may have tolerance to this surface glycoprotein and will not direct an immunological response against it.

Despite the fact that malignant cells may have higher levels of expression for this glycoprotein, it is important to analyze if the animal data demonstrate an immunological response when MaxiVAX is injected. A dose response curve should show that immunological response would increase when the doses are increased. Response should be similar to graft reject or graft versus host disease symptoms to ensure that this vaccine is indeed what it claims to be.

Immunological response should include both humoral and cellular response directed against the MaxiVAX and cells with high levels of the glycoprotein.

10 Immunodiagnostics and Immunoassay

Due to the high specificity and affinity towards antigens, antibodies are ideal tools for the detection and measurement of the presence of antigens in tissues or biological samples. Indeed, during the last two decades, the application of antibodies as powerful analytical agents has greatly facilitated many important developments in biomedical sciences, particularly in endocrinology and neuroscience where most hormones and neuropeptides are present only at minute concentrations in the blood and their quantitative measurements would be virtually impossible without immunoassays. Besides biomedical sciences, immunoassays have also been used in many other areas such as the environmental, forensic, and food sciences. Furthermore, many immunodiagnostic methods have been developed into home testing kits which are sold as the over-the-counter products in drug stores. Therefore, immunodiagnosis and immunodetection have become an important sector in the pharmaceutical industry.

In order to understand the principles and the applications of various immunological techniques, we must first study the interaction between an antibody and an antigen.

Antibody-Antigen Interaction

Affinity and avidity — Spatial complementarity between the structures of an antigen and an antibody has long been considered as the basis of the specificity and affinity of an immunological reaction. The contact areas in antigen and antibody molecules are termed the epitope and paratope, respectively. The close fit between a paratope and an epitope can induce many weak interatomic forces, including hydrophobicity, ionic interaction, hydrogen bonding, and van der Waals' forces. The combination of these forces when acting together is the source of the binding strength between an antibody and an antigen. Since the interaction of antigen and antibody does not involve covalent bond formation, all antibody-antigen interactions, similar to that in enzyme-substrate reactions, are reversible and can be expressed by a simple equilibrium equation:

$$Ag + Ab \rightleftharpoons Ag\text{-}Ab \quad (Ag = antigen; Ab = antibody)$$

or:

$$K = \frac{[Ag\text{-}Ab]}{[Ag] \times [Ab]}$$

where [Ag], [Ab], and [Ag-Ab] are concentrations of antigen, antibody, and antigen-antibody complex, respectively, at equilibrium. The association constant, K, is dependent on the affinity of each individual antibody molecule, and can be as high as 10^{12} M^{-1}. The association constant of an average antigen-antibody interaction is between 10^6 and 10^9 M^{-1}.

The association constant, K, is a measurement of the affinity of a single antigen binding site of an antibody molecule. Almost all antibodies consist of more than two antigen binding sites. In the case of IgM, there are ten binding sites on each immunoglobulin molecule. The multivalent nature can greatly enhance the strength of the binding of an antibody molecule to an antigen with multiple epitopes, and this is referred to as the avidity of the antibody.

Specificity — The specificity of an antibody is determined by the cross-reactivity between the structural analogs of antigen. An antibody is considered highly specific if its binding to the antigen is stronger than to other molecules with similar structures. As shown in Figure 10.1, an antibody raised against a hapten with a structure of A-B-C will have a stronger binding towards the intact structure than the structure of A-B; and A-B, in turn, stronger than A. Therefore, we can say that the antibody is specific to the structure of A-B-C. However, depending on the immunogen, it is possible that a structure of A-B-C-D, which contains a D moiety from the carrier macromolecule as part of the conjugate, will have an even stronger binding to the antibody than the hapten, A-B-C. Therefore, the specificity of an antibody is a relative measurement and the usefulness of an antibody for a specific antigen measurement is dependent on the structures of other substances present in the sample. This is especially important for the measurement of small biological peptides, e.g., neuropeptides, because many of them differ from each other only in one or two amino acids in their structures. This is also true for drugs because drug metabolites may not be distinguish-

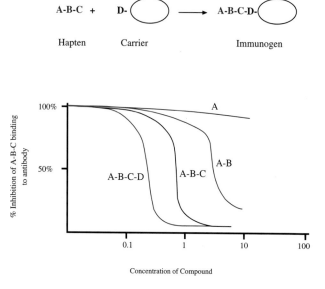

Figure 10.1. The specificity of antibodies. An antibody against the hapten, A-B-C, is prepared by the immunization of animals using a conjugate of A-B-C to a carrier protein as an immunogen. The linkage between A-B-C and the carrier involved a moiety, D, in the structure of the carrier. The relative specificity of the antibody towards A, A-B, A-B-C, and A-B-C-D is determined as the inhibition of the antibody binding of A-B-C. The higher the specificity, the lower the concentration required for the displacement of A-B-C binding, This figure illustrates that the structure of A-B-C-D, due to the similarity to the epitope of the immunogen, has a higher specificity to the anti-A-B-C antibody.

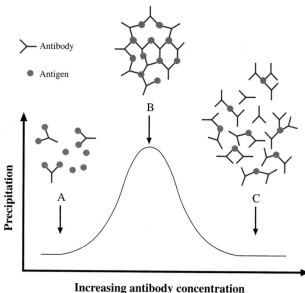

Figure 10.2. The formation of antibody-antigen precipitation. The quantity of the precipitation is determined at a constant antigen concentration with increasing the antibody concentration. At low antibody concentrations (A), no crosslinking between antibody-antigen complexes can be formed; therefore, no precipitation can be detected. At antibody concentrations which are close to the equivalence of the antigen concentration (B), crosslinking of antibody-antigen complexes can be formed; therefore, precipitation is detectable. However, if the antibody concentration is further increased (C), the crosslinking of antibody-antigen complexes become less likely and the amount of precipitation will decrease.

able by the anti-drug antibody which is raised against the structure of drug-macromolecule conjugates. In these cases, before a reliable immunological method can be developed, the specificity of the antibody must be tested for peptide analogs or drug metabolites which possibly are also present in the sample.

Immune precipitation — One of the consequences of the antibody-antigen interaction is the formation of antibody-antigen complex precipitation, i.e., immune precipitins. Immune precipitins are formed due to cross-linking between antibody-antigen complexes. Because antibodies consist of more than two antigen-binding sites, they can serve as a bridge between two antigen molecules. In the case of an antigen molecule possessing two or more epitopes, cross-linking of immune complexes can occur when an equivalent ratio of antibody and antigen concentrations is in the solution. The reaction can be simplified as the following equation:

$$nAg + nAb \underset{k_2}{\overset{k_1}{\rightleftharpoons}} nAg\text{-}Ab \xrightarrow{k_3} (Ag\text{-}Ab)_n \downarrow$$

Generally, $k_1 \gg k_2$ and $k_1 \gg k_3$. Relative to the complex formation, the antibody-antigen precipitation is a very slow process. In addition to the ratio, critical concentrations of antibody and antigen in a solution are also required in order to form the cross-linked complexes, or lattices, large enough to precipitate out from the solution (Figure 10.2). Furthermore, antigens with only one epitope such as haptens or antibodies with only one paratope such as Fab and sFv will not form a precipitate with their corresponding antibodies or antigens.

Detection of Antibody-Antigen Interaction

All immunochemical techniques are based on the interaction between an antigen and an antibody. However, the sensitivity of each technique is dependent on the selected indicator that is labeled on either the antibody, the antigen, or both molecules. Amplification of the signal released from the labeled indicator can further increase the sensitivity of the immunochemical techniques. The following

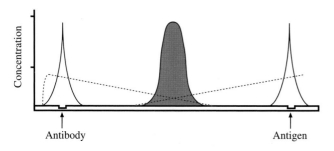

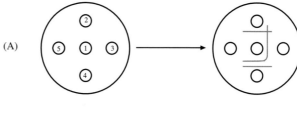

Figure 10.3. The principle of immunodiffusion. Solutions of antibody and antigen are loaded onto two separated spots on a thin slice of gel. As the solutions diffuse along the gel, a concentration gradient will be generated for both the antibody and the antigen (dot-lines). Immune precipitin will form (blue peak) when the two diffusion curves interact at a distance where optimal ratio and concentrations of antibody and antigen can be achieved.

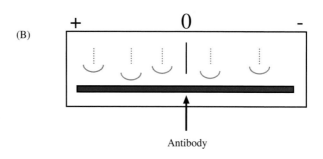

are several examples of the most commonly used methods for the detection of antibody-antigen interaction:

Precipitation: Because of the limitations in the formation of immune precipitins as discussed above, a direct precipitation of antibody-antigen complexes is not a generally useful technique for the detection of antibody-antigen interaction. However, a diffusion of antigen and antibody within a slice of thin gel such as agar or agarose can provide a simple method to detect the immune precipitin formation (Figure 10.3). The diffusion can generate concentration gradients and, therefore, an optimal ratio of antibody and antigen concentrations for the formation of precipitin can be achieved at a distance from the original spot of antigen or antibody in the gel. In addition, both the antigen and the antibody can exist at high concentrations due to the small volume of aqueous phase inside the thin slice of gel matrix; high concentrations of antigen and antibody will favor the formation of precipitation. The immune precipitins in the gel can be observed as white bands or, if the concentration is too low to be seen by the naked eye, can be stained by using protein staining dyes such as Coomassie Blue. Many immunological tests, for example the Ouchterlony test and immunoelectrophoresis (Figure 10.4), are based on the immunodiffusion principle.

Agglutination: When antibodies crosslink on the surface antigens of target cells or antigen-coated particles, an aggregation of particles can be observed which is referred to as agglutination (Figure 10.5). IgM antibodies, by virtue of their multivalent paratopes, are most effective in causing agglutination. Agglutination has been used to detect antibodies against pathogenic cells such as bacteria in patients' blood, for the diagnosis of infectious diseases; most of

Figure 10.4. (A) Ouchterlony test. Antigen and antibody solutions are placed in separated wells in a slice of agar. Immune precipitins form between wells that contain solutions of corresponding antigen and antibody. In this figure, well # 1 contains a mixture of antibodies against antigen-1 and antigen-2. Wells # 2 and 3 contain antigen-1 and -2, respectively. Antigen-1 and -2 are not identical as shown the pattern of crossing precipitin bands. Well # 4 contains a mixture of antigen-1 and -2, as shown two parallel bands with one of the two bands is identical to the antigen in well # 3. Well # 5 contains no antigen-1 or -2 as shown on immune precipitin band formation. (B) Immunoelectrophoresis. A mixture of antigens is first separated in a gel slab by using electrical field, a process called electrophoresis. Depending their charges, antigens will migrate from the original point (0) to either the anode (+) or the cathode (−) with different distance as illustrated in dotted lines in this figure. After the electrophoretic process, a narrow trough is cut along the direction of the electrophoresis migration and an immunodiffusion pattern can be obtained. The appearance as well as the intensity of the precipitin bands can provide information regarding the existence or quantity of certain antigens in the sample such as human serum.

these tests have been replaced by other more sensitive and reliable immunological methods. However, agglutination of microspheres, which can be measured as the change in scattered light due to the increase of particle size, has been used recently to develop commercial immunoassay sys-

(A)

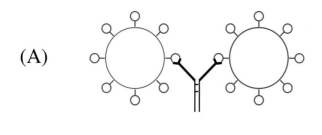

(B)

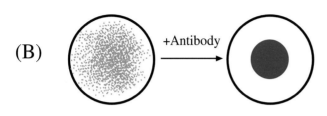

Figure 10.5. (A) Crosslinking of particles can occur when multivalent antibodies against surface antigens are present in the solution. (B) The crosslinking of antigens as shown in (A) can cause the aggregation of antigen-bearing particles, a process which is referred to as agglutination.

tems such as the Quantitative Microsphere System (QMS™, Seradyn). When drug-coated microspheres and a specific anti-drug antibody are used, microsphere agglutination technology can be applied to the quantitative determination of drug concentrations in biological samples.

Fluorescence: Fluorescent labeling is a powerful technique for the detection of antibody binding to antigen, and can be used to detect antigens in biological samples such as cells and tissues. The immunofluorescent staining technique, using fluorescent labeled antibodies, is an important method in histochemistry. Two of the most commonly used fluorescent compounds in antibody labeling are fluorescein isothiocyanate (FITC) and rhodamine isothiocyanate (RITC). Both compounds are easily conjugated to antibodies via amino groups on immunoglobulins. FITC and RITC conjugates displace a green and red fluorescence, respectively, when excited by ultraviolet light. When an immunofluorescent technique is applied to samples with low levels of antigen, an amplification procedure may be used in order to increase the sensitivity; such a procedure is referred to as an indirect immunofluorescence technique (Figure 10.6). Besides increasing the sensitivity, indirect

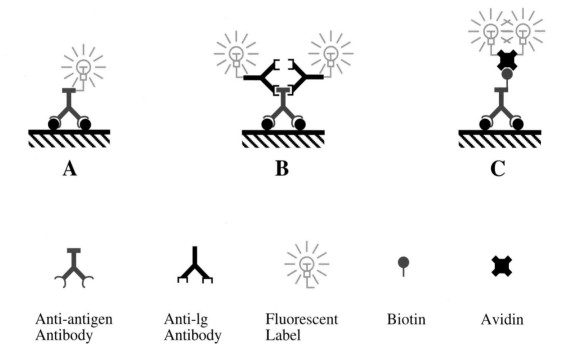

Anti-antigen Antibody

Anti-Ig Antibody

Fluorescent Label

Biotin

Avidin

Figure 10.6. Detection of antibody-antigen binding with fluorescence.
(A) Direct detection: The fluorescent label is directly linked to the anti-antigen antibody. This method, even though it appears to be simple, is less sensitive and involves the conjugation of labels to specific antibodies. (B) and (C) Indirect detection-. Indirect detection methods, such as using fluorescent-labeled anti-immunoglobulins (B) or biotin-avidin system (C). These methods are not only more sensitive than the direct detection method but also can use labeled anti-Ig or labeled avidin as general reagents for fluorescent detection.

Type of immunoassay	Label	Sensitivity (M)
RIA	^{125}I	$10^{-10}-10^{-11}$
IRMA	^{125}I	$10^{-11}-10^{-12}$
ELISA	HRP or AP	$10^{-10}-10^{-11}$
FIA	FITC or RITC	$10^{-9}-10^{-10}$
TFIA	Eu-chelates	$10^{-12}-10^{-13}$
LIA	acridinium ester	$10^{-11}-10^{-12}$
Energy-transfer LIA	luminol and FITC	$10^{-12}-10^{-13}$

Table 10.1. Comparison of the sensitivity of selected immunoassay techniques.

immunofluorescence uses a fluorescent anti-immuno-globulin antibody as a general fluorescent reagent for different antigen-antibody systems, and therefore, the labeling of the specific antibody for each specific immunodetection procedure can be avoided.

Radioisotopes: Radioisotope-labeled antigen or antibody can provide a very sensitive method for the detection of antibody-antigen interactions (Table 10.1). Many radioisotopes such as ^{125}I, ^{3}H, and ^{14}C have been used for both *in vitro* and *in vivo* detection of immune complexes. For *in vivo* diagnostic applications, such as the use of anti-tumor antibodies for tumor detection in cancer patients and anti-fibrin antibodies for blood clot localization in stroke patients, the location of gamma emitter-labeled antibodies inside body tissues can be detected by means of a gamma-ray scanner.

Enzymes: Enzymes can be used to label an antibody for detecting immune complex formation by measuring the specific enzymatic reaction. Because an enzyme usually has a very fast turnover rate, i.e., the rate of converting substrates to products, an enzymatic reaction can be also considered as an amplifier in itself and, when conjugated to antibodies, can provide a very sensitive measurement of antibody-antigen complex formation. One of the many advantages of using enzymes as indicators is that many enzyme reactions can generate colored products and therefore the enzyme reaction can be observed visually; this is important for the development of home-diagnostic kits when the result from the assay can be evaluated only by the naked eye. Two of the most commonly used enzymes are horse-radish peroxidase (HPO) and alkaline phosphatase (AP).

As shown in the following two equations, substrates can be selected that will generate colored products for visual detection:

$$H_2O_2 + \text{reduced TMB} \xrightarrow{\text{HPO}} H_2O + \text{oxidized TMB}$$
$$\text{(Colorless)} \qquad\qquad \text{(Yellow, 450nm)}$$

$$\text{p-Nitrophenyl phosphate} \xrightarrow{\text{AP}} \text{p-Nitrophenol + Phosphate}$$
$$\text{(Colorless)} \qquad\qquad \text{(Yellow, 440 nm)}$$

Other methods: There are many other methods that have been used for the detection of antibody-antigen interactions. Using electron-dense labels such as ferritin, a protein with a large iron core, the binding of an antibody to the tissue or cell antigen can be detected using electron microscopic techniques. Other labels include chemiluminescent or bioluminescent compounds which can generate light with specific wavelengths upon chemical or biochemical treatment. One modification of chemiluminescent detection of antibody-antigen interactions is to use the phenomenon of energy transfer (Figure 10.7). In this case both antigen and antibody molecules will be modified, one with a fluorescent group and the other with a luminescent group. Upon excitation by chemical or biochemical reactions, the luminescent groups will transfer the energy to the fluorescent groups within an antibody-antigen complex due to the proximity of the two groups. Consequently, the emission wavelength of the complex will be different from that of the unbound antibodies or antigens, and therefore the antibody-antigen interaction can be detected. Similarly, when the antigen and the antibody molecules are modified with a fluorescent group and a quencher, respectively, the antibody-antigen interaction can be detected as a decrease in the fluorescence intensity.

Principles of Immunoassays

Methods which use antibodies as analytical reagents for the quantitative measurement of antigen concentrations in samples are referred to as immunoassays. Although uncommon, immunoassays can also be used for the quantitative measurement of antibody concentrations in physiological fluids. In all immunoassays, the principle of the methodology is the detection of antibody-antigen complexes; the method of detection used is generally the name of the immunoassay technique. For example, if a radioactive isotope is used for the detection of antibody-antigen complexes, the method is called radioimmunoassay (RIA). Similarly, if an enzyme or a fluorescent reagent is used, the method is called enzyme immunoassay (EIA) or fluorescence immunoassay (FIA), respectively.

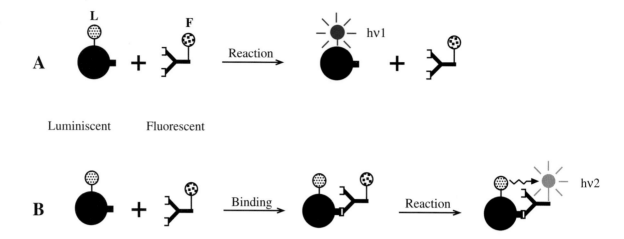

Luminiscent   Fluorescent

Figure 10.7. Energy-transfer fluorescence technology. An example is illustrated in this figure in which an antigen and an antibody are labeled with luminescent (L) and fluorescent (F) labels, respectively. Without immune complex formation, the mixture will responds to the luminescent excitation such as a chemical (chemiluminescent) or a biochemical (bioluminescent) reaction to release a phosphorescent light with a wavelength (hv1). However, with the formation of immune complexes, the fluorescent group is brought to a close proximity of the luminescent group and, when exposed to the exciting condition, the energy from the luminescent group can be transferred to the fluorescent group. Consequently, a fluorescent light with a longer wavelength (hv2) can be detected. By measuring the specific hv2 wavelength intensity, the amount of immune complex can be determined in the presence of free antigen or antibody in the solution.

Besides the detection method, immunoassays can be classified by the principle of the quantitative measurement as competitive and non-competitive. In competitive immunoassays, antigen molecules in the sample compete with a constant quantity of labeled antigen molecules to a limited number of antigen-binding sites of antibody molecules. When the signal from the labeled antigen in the antigen-antibody complex (such as the radioactivity) is measured, it decreases as the concentration of antigen in the sample increases. The extent of decreasing labeled antigen binding is compared with a standard curve to determine the concentration of antigen in the sample (Figure 10.8). In non-competitive immunoassays, the antigen molecules in the sample are captured by an excess of antibodies which usually are immobilized on the surface of a matrix. The captured antigen molecules can be detected by using a labeled second antibody which recognizes different epitopes on the antigen (Figure 7.9). Therefore, the first antibody is referred to as a capturing antibody while the second antibody is a signal antibody. Non-competitive immunoassays are also called immunometric assays. For example, non-competitive radioimmunoassay is called immunoradiometric assay (IRMA). Generally, in non-competitive immunoassays, the antigen concentrations are proportional to the signal detected from the second antibody (Figure 10.9). Therefore, for the measurement of antigen at low concentrations, non-competitive immunoassays are more accurate than their corresponding competitive methods.

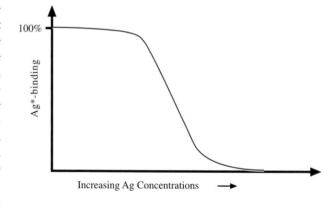

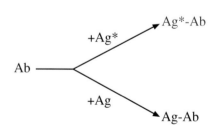

Figure 10.8. Competitive immunoassay — Unlabeled antigen molecules (Ag) compete with labeled antigens (Ag*) for a limited number of antibody binding sites (Ab). The binding of labeled Ag* to Ab decreases as the concentration of antigen increases.

136

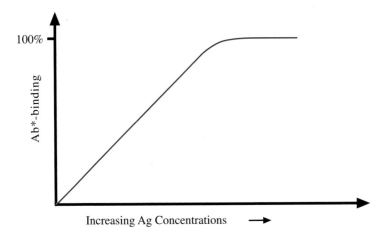

$$\mathbf{Ag} \quad + \quad \mathbf{Ab} \longrightarrow \mathbf{Ab\text{-}Ag} \quad + \quad \mathbf{Ab^*} \longrightarrow \mathbf{Ab\text{-}Ag\text{-}Ab^*}$$

Figure 10.9. Non-competitive immunoassay _ Antigen molecules (Ag) bind to an unlabeled antibody (Ab), and a second antibody with label (Ab*) recognizes a different epitope on Ag and forms a ternary complex, Ab-Ag-Ab*. The binding of labeled Ab* to Ag-Ab complexes increases as the concentration of antigen increases; therefore, the non-competitive immunoassay is more sensitive than its competitive counterpart.

Another important step in most immunoassay procedures is the separation of antibody-antigen complexes from the free antibody and antigen molecules. As shown in Figures 10.8 and 10.9, the unbound labeled antigen or antibody must be removed in order to measure the amount of antibody-antigen complex. One of the most commonly used techniques for the separation of free antigen from antibody-bound antigen is the second antibody precipitation method. In a competitive immunoassay, because of the low concentrations of both antibody and antigen, antibody-antigen complexes do not form a precipitation spon-

taneously. Therefore, in order to obtain a precipitation, a relatively large amount of non-specific immunoglobulin from the same species of the anti-antigen antibody and a second antibody which is raised against the first antibody immunoglobulin must be added to the immunoassay solution after the incubation of the radioactive antigen, the antibody and the sample. Such a precipitation will consist mostly of the second antibody-immunoglobulin complexes with the coprecipitated antigen-antibody complexes but not the unbound antigen (Figure 10.10).

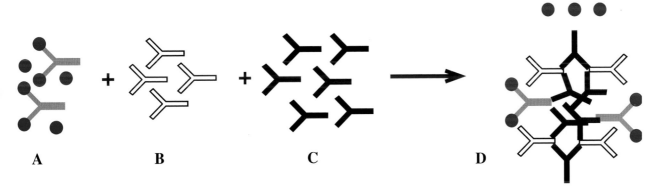

Figure 10.10. Double-antibody technique for the precipitation of antigen-antibody complexes. Homologous immunoglobulin (B) is added to the immune complexes (A) as carriers and, subsequently, an anti-immunoglobulin antibody raised from a different species is added as the second antibody (C). Immune precipitin is formed (D) which will co-precipitate the antigen-antibody complexes but not free antigen molecules.

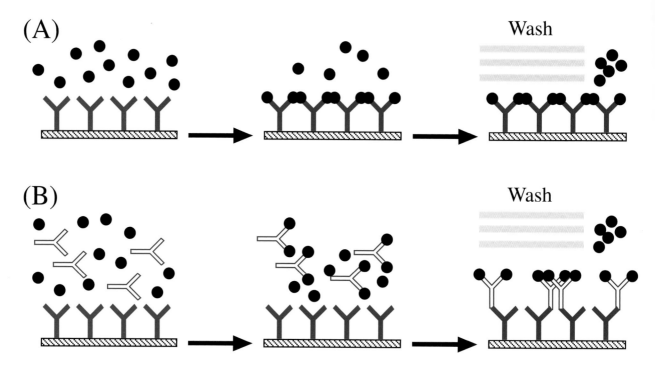

Figure 10.11. Separation of antigen-antibody complexes from free antigen molecules using immobilized antibodies. (A) Immobilization of anti-antigen antibodies. (B) Immobilization of anti-immunoglobulin antibodies to capture antigen-antibody complexes. In both cases, free antigen molecules can be removed from the antibody-bound antigens by washing the surface of the immobilizing matrix.

Other methods that can separate immune complexes from free antigen or antibody include the immobilization of antibody on the surface of a matrix such as beads and test tubes. In this case, unbound antigens can be easily washed away (Figure 10.11). When immunoassays are used to determine the concentrations of small molecular haptens in samples, the free haptens usually can be removed from antibody-bound haptens by using absorbent materials such charcoal and membranes. Organic solvents, e.g., ethanol or polyethylene glycol, can also be used to precipitate antibody-hapten complexes while keeping the unbound haptens in solution.

When an immunoassay procedure requires separation of the unbound antigen or antibody from the immune complexes, it is referred to as a heterogeneous immunoassay. Most commonly used immunoassays are heterogeneous immunoassays. However, if an immunoassay procedure can measure the antibody-antigen complexes without separating the unbound antigen or antibody, it will not only save time and expense, but also avoid the separation procedures. Immunoassays which do not require a separation step are referred to as homogeneous immunoassays and are highly desirable for the development of simple or automated immunoassay systems.

Examples of Immunoassays

Radioimmunoassays: Radioimmunoassays, including both competitive (RIA) and non-competitive (IRMA) methods (Figures 10.8 and 10.9), were the earliest immunoassay techniques developed. In RIA, antigens in the sample compete with radiolabeled antigens for binding to limited binding sites in the antibody. After the separation of unbound antigens, the amount of radioactivity in the antigen-antibody complex can be measured and the amount of antigen in the sample can be determined. RIA can be applied to both macromolecular antigens and small molecular haptens. In immunoradiometric assay (IRMA), a non-competitive procedure, radioactive isotopes are coupled to the second signal antibody and, therefore, can be applied only to antigens with multiple epitopes. Despite their simplicity and sensitivity, radioimmunoassays have many practical disadvantages. First, counting radioactivity not only needs expensive equipment but also is very time consuming. Second, radioisotope-labeled antigens are not always available and some isotopes have very short half-lives ($t_{1/2}$), e.g., $t_{1/2}$ for ^{125}I is only 60 days. The most serious problem facing the practice of radioimmunoassay is the potential health hazard of the radiation, and, consequently, the problem in the

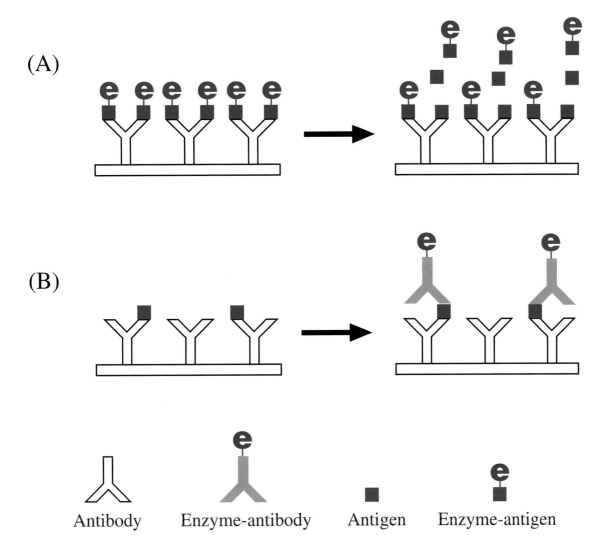

(A)

(B)

Antibody   Enzyme-antibody   Antigen   Enzyme-antigen

Figure 10.12. Comparison of (A) competitive and (B) non-competitive enzyme immunoassays. In competitive enzyme immunoassays, the enzyme is conjugated to the antigen which competes unlabeled antigen to the binding of the immobilized antibody. After removal of free conjugates by washing, the enzyme activity associated with the immobilized antibody is measured and a competition curve can be obtained which is similar to the standard curve as shown in Figure 10.8. In non-competitive enzyme immunoassays, the enzyme is conjugated to a second antibody which recognizes the epitope of an antigen differed from the immobilized first antibody; therefore, the non-competitive immunoassays are also known as the "sandwich" methods. After the removal of the free enzyme conjugates, the enzyme activity associated with the immobilized antibody is measured and a linear antigen-dependent curve is obtained which is similar to that in Figure 10.9.

disposal of radioactive waste. Therefore, immunoassay techniques using non-isotope labels are more desirable for general applications.

Enzyme immunoassays: As described in the Principles of Immunoassays, enzymes can provide a sensitivity comparable to radioisotopes due to the high turnover rate. In most EIA procedures, the antibody is first immobilized on the surface of a matrix such as polystyrene or polyacrylamide plates. Such a procedure is also known as enzyme labeled

immunosorbent assay (ELISA). ELISA can be either a competitive or a non-competitive method (Figure 10.12). Since multiwell plastic plates, such as 96-well plates, can be used as the absorbent matrix for the immobilization of capturing antibodies, a large number of samples can be tested at one time. In addition, the enzymatic reactions can be monitored using a microtiter plate reader, which simultaneously scans the optical absorption of all 96 wells; therefore, ELISA can be a much faster procedure than RIA. Even though enzymes are superior to radioisotopes in terms of

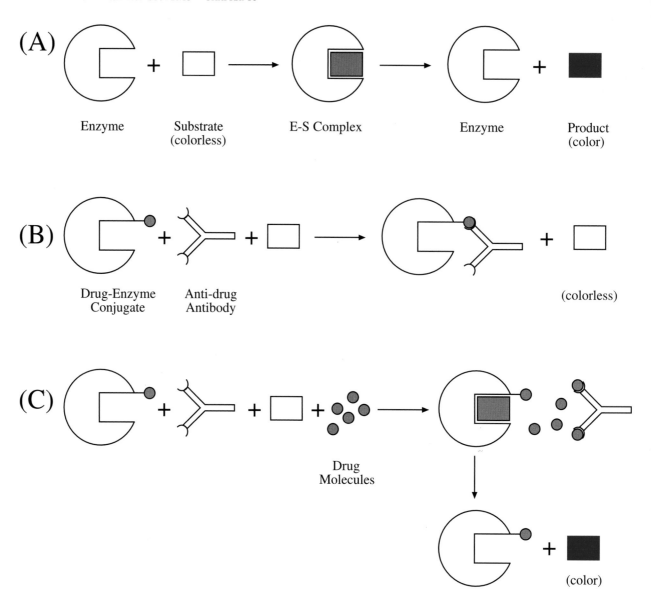

Figure 10.13. Enzyme-multiplied immunoassay test (EMIT™). (A) An enzyme system is selected which can convert a colorless substrate to a colored product; hence, the enzyme reaction can be monitored by the color formation. (B) A hapten (such as a drug) is conjugated to the enzyme at a position close to the active site. When the antibody to the hapten binds to the hapten moiety on the enzyme-hapten conjugate, it will block the accessibility of substrate to the active site and, therefore, there will be no colored product formation. (C) When a sample is added to the system, the free hapten molecules in the sample will compete with the enzyme-hapten conjugate to the antibody binding and prevent the blockage of the active site of the enzyme. The enzyme activity can be recovered as indicated by the formation of a color product which is proportional to the concentration of hapten in the sample. Please notice that in this immunoassay technique no separation of free hapten and antibody-bound hapten is required. Therefore, EMIT™ is a homogeneous immunoassay.

health hazards, they suffer from instability and potential inhibition by components present in biological samples. Nevertheless, ELISA is currently the most commonly used technique in immunoassay.

In addition to ELISA, which is still a heterogeneous immunoassay, several homogeneous immunoassay procedures have been developed by using enzymes as indicators.

One homogeneous enzyme immunoassay is the Enzyme-Multiplied Immunoassay Test (EMIT™, Syva-Syntex) (Figure 10.13). In this method, small molecules such as drugs are coupled to an enzyme. When an anti-hapten antibody binds to the enzyme-hapten conjugate, the enzymatic activity is altered, or more likely inhibited. The inhibitory effect of the antibody on the enzymatic activity of the enzyme-hapten conjugate is reversed by free hapten molecules present in the sample. Therefore, the higher the hapten concentration in the assay solution, the higher the measured enzyme activity. EMIT™ is usually used for the detection of small molecular drugs, while ELISA, a heterogeneous immunoassay technique, is usually used for the detection of macromolecular antigens such as proteins or polypeptide hormones.

Another example of homogeneous enzyme immunoassay is the Cloned Enzyme Donor Immunoassay (CEDIA™, Microgenics). In CEDIA™, recombinant DNA technology is used to generate two polypeptides (a large one, the acceptor or EA, and a small one, the donor or ED) from the β-galactosidase gene. Spontaneous association of these two polypeptides can produce an active enzyme β-galactosidase. A hapten molecule can be linked to ED and anti-hapten antibody can prevent the formation of the active enzyme from EA and hapten-ED. In the presence of free hapten molecules, hapten-ED will be displaced from the binding to antibody and thus active enzyme can be regenerated. Similar to EMIT™, CEDIA™ is also used for the detection of small molecular drugs only.

Fluorescent immunoassays: Because of the limited sensitivity of the instrumentation as well as the high background of fluorescent substances present in biological samples, conventional FIA are not generally practical as an immunodiagnostic technique. However, several companies have developed techniques, such as polarized fluorescent immunoassays (PFIA) and time-resolved fluorescence immunoassays (TFIA), which can distinguish the sample's fluorescence from the background fluorescence by the difference in their decay rates. One of the most successful fluorescence immunoassays is the use of europium chelated labels. Fluorescent europium chelates possess many unique characteristics, including their fluorescence half-lives being about ten thousand-fold longer than those of conventional fluorophores. This makes the rare-earth metal ion complexes ideal labels for the development of sensitive TFIA. Furthermore, as described previously (Figure 10.7), fluorescence when combined with either luminescence or quenching groups can be a very sensitive method to detect antigen-antibody interaction upon energy transfer or quenching between the two labeled groups. Such a system has been used for developing homogeneous immunoassays with high sensitivities, e.g Fluorescence Energy Transfer Immunoassay (FETI).

Commercial Immunodiagnostic Kits

Immunodiagnostic kits, together with other home testing products, represent one of the most rapidly growing products in the market of pharmacy. It is postulated that, in the year 2000, all households in the U.S. will regularly use at least one home testing product. The rapid expansion of the home testing product market is due to many reasons, such as the increase in self-awareness of one's health, the better understanding of etiology of many diseases, the expense and inconvenience of hospital visits, and the change of health insurance policies in many developed countries. In addition, one of the most important factors for the commercialization of home diagnostic systems is the advance of biotechnological industries. Home testing kits must be easy to use by a person with no training and experience; their results must be simple, yet reliable, in interpretation. Immunoassay can fulfill all of these criteria and is one of the most popular techniques that has been used in the development of home diagnostic systems.

Because it is low in toxicity, easy in interpretation, and high in sensitivity, enzyme immunoassay has advantages over other immunological methods for the development of home testing kits. For example, over-the-counter pregnancy test kits are mostly based on the principle of ELISA applied to human chorionic gonadotropin (hCG), a glycoprotein hormone normally produced by the placenta during pregnancy. A significant increase of hCG in the urine of women can be detected by ELISA at only 4 to 5 days after conception. The hCG molecule consists of two subunits, i.e., α- and β-hCG. The α-subunit is more or less identical to many hormones while the β-subunit is unique to hCG. Therefore, antibodies against the β-subunit of hCG are used in developing specific immunodiagnostic kits for the pregnancy test. Other antigens that have been used for the development of home testing kits include luteinizing hormone (LH) for the determination of ovulation time in women and the streptococcus antigen for the detection of strep throat.

Types of Immunodiagnostic Kits

TEST TUBE TYPE

The immunodiagnostic kits using test tubes are the prototypes of immunoassay kits, and many of them are still on the market but they are mostly used in laboratories. A test tube type kit usually consists of many test tubes and small vials of reagents. The test tubes are coated with the capturing antibody (Figure 10.14). When a sample such as urine is added to the tube, antigens in the sample will be bound by the immobilized antibody. After the tubes have been rinsed by either water or the supplied buffer in the kit, a solution of signalling antibody which is a conjugate of enzyme-antibody, is added to the tubes. After being maintained at room temperature for a short period of time, the tubes are rinsed again and an enzyme assay solution from the kit added to each tube. Color develops in the tubes on enzymatic reaction, and the intensity of the color can be used to determine the concentration of antigen in each sample.

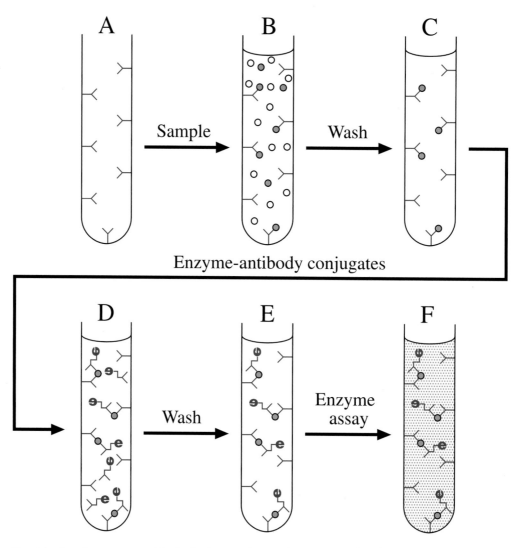

Figure 10.14. Test-tube type immunoassay kit: Antibody-coated test tube (A) is incubated with sample solution (B). Antigen molecules in the sample will bind to immobilized antibodies, and other molecules will be washed off (C). Enzyme conjugates of a second antibody will be added to the tube (D) and, after the second wash, only antigen-bound enzyme-antibody conjugates will be present in the tube (E). The amount of antibody-bound antigen can be determined by the measurement of the enzymatic activity in the tube.

One of the advantages of the test tube type kit is that it can be used to determine a large number of samples at the same time. In addition, with a simple instrument such as a colorimeter and some standard samples, test tube kits can produce quantitative measurement of the antigen; this may be more useful than qualitative detection for the diagnosis of certain diseases. However, in order to give an optimal result, some basic handling techniques may be required, and these may not be as easy to apply to home testing kits. Furthermore, because of the complications of enzyme kinetics, reactions in test tubes must be terminated at the same time by treatment (such as acidification) in order to compare the color. The kit should be stored properly, generally in a refrigerator but not a freezer, and should be discarded after the expiration date. Unused tubes or solutions should not be saved for future use and reagents from different kits should not be mixed. To avoid problems associated with handling and storage, most kits contain positive and negative controls. In this case, an assay result is reliable only if both positive and negative tubes show expected results.

COATED DIP-STICK TYPE

In dip-stick type kits, the capturing antibodies are coated on the surface of a plastic stick at one end (Figure 10.15).

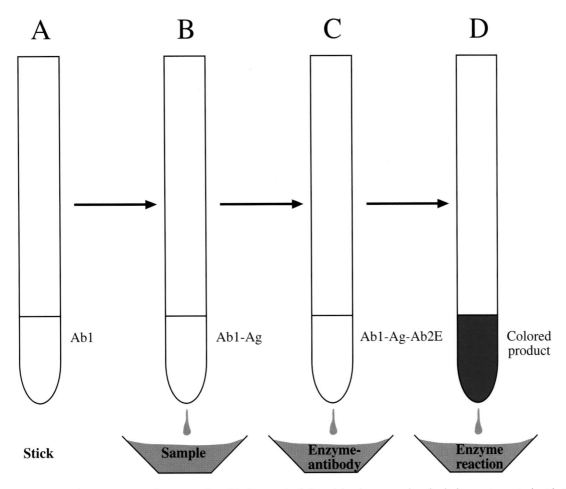

Figure 10.15. Dip-stick type immunodiagnostic kit: (A) One end of the stick, shown as the shaded area, is coated with the capturing antibody (Ab1). (B) When this antibody-coated end is dipped into a sample solution, antigen molecules in the sample will be bound by the immobilized antibodies (Ab1 -Ag). (C) After extensive rinsing, the stick is then dipped into a solution containing enzyme-antibody conjugates (Ab2-E) which recognize epitopes different from that of the capturing antibodies on the surface of the same antigen molecule. (D) After extensively rinsing to remove free conjugates, the enzyme activity retained on the stick is detected by dipping into an enzyme substrate solution which will generate a color product on the stick. Therefore, the appearance of color on the stick indicates a positive result of the assay.

This stick is dipped into a sample, rinsed and then dipped into a solution of the enzyme-antibody conjugate as the signalling antibody. Finally, after rinsing extensively to remove unbound enzyme-antibody, the stick is dipped into a solution for the enzymatic assay. The appearance of a color at the antibody-coated end of the stick indicates a positive result. Some of the dip-stick type kits also provide a color chart which can be used as a semi-quantitative estimation for the antigen concentrations by the comparison of the color intensity.

The dip-stick type kits are easy to use but they still contain solutions and they must be stored properly. Some dip-stick kits include a positive control in the same stick, and the result is considered to be positive only if the control

area on the same stick also shows the color. Because the production of the dip-stick type immunoassay kits is easy and low-cost, currently this type is the most commonly used technique in the development of the over-the-counter home testing kits.

FLOW-THROUGH TYPE

Flow-through type immunoassay kits consist of three vials of solutions, i.e., a solution of the enzyme-antibody conjugate, a solution of enzyme substrates, and a solution of washing buffer, and a test disc (Figure 10.16). In the center of the disc, there is an opening which is covered by a filter with thick absorbent pad underneath. On the filter, two

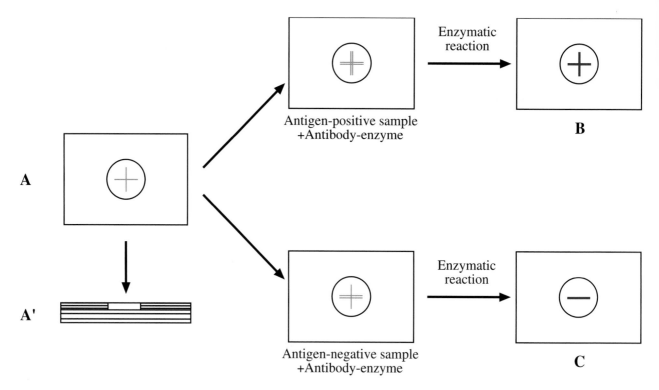

Figure 10.16. Flow-through type immunodiagnostic kit. A flow-through type immunodiagnostic kit, such as Abbott Laboratories' TestPack™, contains a disc (A) with a window opening at the center which is covered with a layer of membrane. On the membrane, an anti-antigen antibody is immobilized as a vertical line, and the antigen is immobilized as a horizontal line. A thick layer of an absorbent material is placed underneath the membrane in the disc (A'). When an antigen-positive solution is added to the disc and washed, followed by the addition of an anti-antigen antibody-enzyme conjugate, both the horizontal and the vertical lines will bind the enzyme conjugate. After the addition of enzyme assay solution to the disc, color will be developed in both lines as a positive sign (B). When an antigen-negative sample is added to the disc, followed by the addition of the anti-antigen antibody-enzyme conjugate, only the horizontal line will bind the enzyme conjugate, and therefore, color will appear only in the horizontal line as a negative line (C).

reagents are immobilized to form two lines, one is the capturing antibody and the other is the antigen or the anti-enzyme-antibody conjugate. This two lines can be arranged in different patterns, e.g., as a cross. When a sample contains no antigen, only one line, or a "−" sign, will show color; on the other hand, if a sample contains antigen, both lines, or a "+" sign, will show the color. Therefore, in this type of immunodiagnostic kit, one of the two signs must appears on the test disc; otherwise, the result of the assay is invalid.

LATERAL FLOW TYPE

This type of immunoassay kit is derived from the flow-through type with two important modifications. First, the sample solution is spotted directly at one end of an absorbent strip and the solution migrates towards the other end via the capillary phenomenon. Second, the signalling antibody usually is not an enzyme conjugate, but rather a colored antibody such as the colloidal gold antibody complexes. When the sample migrates along the strip, it first encounters the signalling antibody and antigen-antibody complexes will be formed. These soluble complexes further migrate until they are captured by the immobilized anti-antigen antibody on the strip. The capturing of the antigen-antibody complexes will concentrate the colloidal gold to a small area and a color band will be observed (Figure 10.17). Similar to the flow-through type of assay kits, a line of immobilized anti-signalling antibody can be used after the capturing antibody line, and this line is used to confirm the negative result. One of the advantages of the lateral flow type of immunoassay kit over other types of kits is that the lateral type kits need only a test disc, but not other reagents or solutions. Therefore, a lateral flow type can save in production costs, overcome the storage problems, and minimize the mistakes in following the instructions in the kit. Several of the recent over-the-counter diagnostic kits, e.g Warner-Lambert's e.p.t.™ Preg-

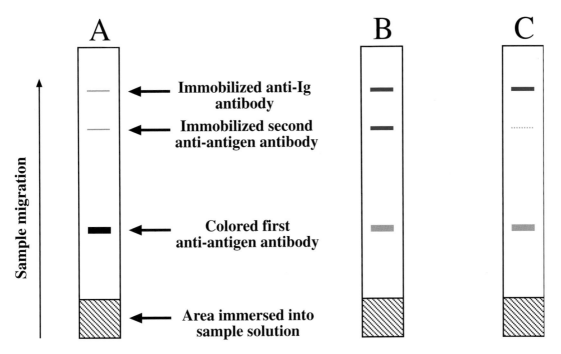

Figure 10.17. Lateral flow type immunodiagnostic kit: A lateral flow type immunodiagnostic kit consists of a strip which has been treated with three different types of antibodies. As shown in (A), the first one is a colored anti-antigen antibody (such as anti-antigen antibody-colloidal gold conjugate) which is precoated but not immobilized on the strip. Above this preloaded colored antibody, there are two immobilized bands of antibodies; one is the immobilized second anti-antigen antibody and the other is the immobilized anti-immunoglobulin antibody. When the designated end of the trip is immersed into the sample such as the urine, the solution will migrate upward by the capillary action. The solution will first encounter the colored anti-antigen antibody and, if the solution contains antigen, soluble antibody-antigen complexes will be formed. The soluble complexes will continue to migrate until they are captured by the immobilized second anti-antigen antibody to form an intensive color band. The excess of colored antibody which contains no antigen will further migrate and captured by the anti-immunoglobulin antibody to form a second colored band, and therefore, two bands will show up to give a positive result (B). In antigen-negative samples, only the second band will show up (C). Therefore, in using this type of immunodiagnostic kit, e.g. Warner-Lambert's e.p.t. Pregnancy Test, two color lines indicate a positive result, and one color line indicates a negative result. If none of the two bands show up, the assay is invalid. In Abbott's TestPack+Plus kits, the two lines of immobilized antibodies are arranged to cross each other, and therefore, a "+" or "−" sign indicates a positive or negative result, respectively.

nancy Test and Abbott's TestPack+Plus™, are based on the lateral flow technology.

Advantages and Limitations of Immunodiagnostic Kits

In this chapter, we have discussed several examples of immunoassay techniques. It should be emphasized that there are many other immunological methods that have been developed or are still being developed. Many of them may enter the market as immunodiagnostic kits in the near future.

However, there are several inherent limitations when using an immunoassay kit in home diagnosis. First, an immunoassay measures only the concentration of an antigen. It is possible that an increase of an antigen concentration can be a result of many other physiological or pathological conditions. For example, the increase of hCG concentration in the urine, as detected by pregnancy test kits, could be due to trophoblastic disease and not pregnancy. For infectious diseases, an immunoassay kit mostly measures only a specific bacterial or viral antigen; it may fail to detect mutants from the original pathogens. Furthermore, substances cross-reacting with the antibody or antigen-positive dead bacteria may give a false positive result. When enzyme immunoassay procedures are used, substances present in a biological sample, which could be either inhibitors or activators of the enzyme, may produce false positive or negative results. For over-the-counter immunodiagnostic kits, it is important that the instructions for both the use and the storage of the kit should be followed carefully. Conditions for storage of these products, particularly the temperature, are critical for the activities of both enzyme and antibody, because they are proteins and are subject to denaturation by high temperature, U.V. light, oxidation, and high humidity. Shelf-lives of reagent solutions in the kits should be checked before use. Human error in following the instructions may also be the reason for the failure of home diagnostic kits. ∎

References

- **Colbert DL.** (1994). Drug abuse screening with immunoassays: unexpected cross-reactivities and other pitfalls. *Br J Biomed Sci,* **51,** 136–146

- **Ekins RP.** (1993). New perspectives in radioimmunoassay. *Nucl Med Commun,* **14,** 721–735

- **Gosling JP, Basso LV, eds.** (1994). *Immunoassay – Lab Anal Clinl Appl.* Boston: Butterworth–Heineman

- **Hage DS.** (1995). Immunoassays. *Anal Chem,* **67,** 455R–462R

- **Ngo TT, ed.** (1988). *Nonisotopic Immunoassay.* New York, New York: Plenum Press

- **Price CP, Newman DJ, eds.** (1991). *Principles and Practice of Immunoassay.* New York, New York: Macmillan Publishers

- **Rongen HA, Hoetelmans RM, Bult A, Van Bennekom WP.** (1994). Chemiluminescence and immunoassays. *J Pharm Biomed Anal,* **12,** 433–462

Self-Assessment Questions

Question 1: One of your patients has purchased from your pharmacy an immune-based diagnostic kit testing for the "strep-throat." One week later, she came back and complained that the kit indicated that her son had a strep-throat; yet, a subsequent laboratory culture test from a hospital showed a negative result. How can you explain this discrepancy between the two tests?

Question 2: RH is a recently divorced man whose ex-wife has been diagnosed with human immunodeficiency virus (HIV) infection. When RH became aware of his ex-wife's HIV status, he too was tested for HIV in a hospital laboratory using an immunoassay method and was found to be HIV-negative. One year later, he was admitted to hospital because of respiratory illness and dramatic weight loss. The HIV-test remained negative. However, other laboratory tests confirmed the presence of Pneumocystis carinii pneumonia, and a CD4+ count of 129 cells/mL (CD4+ <200 is a diagnosis of AIDS).
What are possible explanations for the discrepancies between those tests?

Answer 1: There are several possible explanations for this discrepancy between the immunodiagnostic kit and the laboratory culture test. First, the immunodiagnostic kit measures only the antigen, while culture tests detect only intact and living bacteria. Therefore, it is possible that immunodiagnostic kit can not detect antigen-negative mutants. However, in this case, the immunodiagnotic kit actually produced a positive result while the culture test was negative. This may be due to the presence of dead bacteria in the throat sample, which could result from taking medicine before the test and would not be detectable in the culture test. However, human errors can include contamination, reagent kit expiration, and incorrect sample processing.

Answer 2: Currently HIV infection is screened by using enzyme-linked immunosorbent assays (ELISA) in clinical laboratories to detect the presence of antibodies directed against HIV antigens. However, there were reports that negative results were observed in patients who have confirmed HIV infection. RH apparently had already developed a full-blown AIDS syndrome, but was HIV-negative in both tests. Several factors may contribute to false negative results of the test:

1. Following HIV infection, there is a lag period where antibody production is below detectable range of the test kits. This period of time is referred to as the "window period." RH's first test was performed possibly during the window period.

2. Persistent negative results may be obtained if infections with divergent HIV strains of different antigens, such as HIV-2 which is prevalent in Africa. RH may carry a mutant of HIV, which has alternated antigen for the ELISA assay.

3. In rare cases, HIV-infected patients who are initially HIV seropositive may become seronegative, i.e., the lack of detectable anti-HIV antibody in patient's blood samples. This change is called "serorevert", and is possibly due to the deterioration of humoral immunity in AIDS patients.

Appendices — Immunological Agents as Therapeutic Drugs

Product Description	Trade Name	Indication	Company (Partner)	Status
IL-2 (Aldeskine)	Proleukin	Metastatic renal cell carcinoma	Chiron	Market
IL-2 (Aldeskine)	Proleukin	Ovarian cancer	Chiron	Phase II/III
IL-2 (Aldeskine)	Proleukin	Malignant melanoma	Chiron	Phase II
rhIL-2 (Aldeskine)	Proleukin	Metastatic renal cell carcinoma	Ligand (Chiron)	Market
rhIL-2 gene therapy	—	Renal cell cancer and malignant melanoma	Transkaryotic Therapies	Phase I
IL-2 + Indinavir	Proleukin	HIV/AIDS	Chiron	Phase II
IL-2	Proleukin	HIV/AIDS	Chiron	Phase II
IL-2 + CenTNF	Proleukin	HIV/AIDS	Chiron	Phase II
DAB 389 (IL-2 fusion protein)	—	HIV/AIDS	Seragen	Phase I/II
rhIL-3	—	Cancer-related blood cell deficiencies	Genetics Institute (Norvatis)	Phase III
rhIL-6	—	Platelet restoration (thrombocytopenia)	Genetics Institute (Norvatis)	Phase II/III
rhIL-11	Neumega	Inflammatory bowel disease	Genetics Institute	Phase III
rhIL-11	Neumega	Platelet restoration (thrombocytopenia)	Genetics Institute	Market
rhIL-11	Neumega	PBPC mobilization	Genetics Institute	Phase II
rhIL-11	Neumega	Chemotherapy-induced mucositis	Genetics Institute	Phase I/II
rhIL-12 (NKSF)	—	Cancer	Genetics Institute (Wyeth Ayerst)	Phase I/II
rhIL-12 (NKSF)	—	HIV/AIDS	Genetics Institute (Wyeth Ayerst)	Phase I/II
rhIL-12 (NKSF)	—	HIV-infection	Genetics Institute (Wyeth Ayerst)	Phase I

Appendix 1. Interleukins.

Product Description	Trade Name	Indication	Company (Partner)	Status
r-huEPO	Epogen	End-stage renal disease anemia	Amgen	Marketed
r-huEPO	Procrit	Anemia associated with AIDS therapies	Amgen (Johnson & Johnson)	Marketed
r-huEPO	Procrit	Chemo-assoc. anemia in non-myeloid malignancies	Amgen (Johnson & Johnson)	Marketed
r-huEPO	Epogen	Kidney dialysis patients (raise hematocrits)	Amgen	Phase II
r-huG-CSF	Neupogen	Pneumonia sepsis	Amgen	Phase III
r-huG-CSF	Neupogen	Multilobar pneumonia	Amgen	Phase III
r-huG-CSF	Neupogen	Adjunct to chemotherapy	Amgen	Market
r-huG-CSF	Neupogen	Febrile neutropenia post-high-dose chemo.	Amgen	Market
r-huG-CSF	Neupogen	Severe chronic neutropenia	Amgen	Market
r-huG-CSF	Neupogen	Allogeneic or autologous BMT engraftment or failure	Amgen	Market
r-huG-CSF	Neupogen	Mobilization of autologous PBPCs post-chemo.	Amgen	Market
r-huG-CSF	Neupogen	Acute myeloid leukemia (AML)	Amgen	Market
r-huG-CSF	Neupogen	Neutropenia associated with AIDS therapies	Amgen	Market
r-huG-CSF	Neupogen	Head Injury	Amgen	Market
r-huG-CSF	Neupogen	Neonatal sepsis	Amgen	Phase III
rhGM-CSF	Leucomax	Low white blood cell counts	Genetics Institute (Schering-Plough/Norvatis)	Appr. Europe
GM-CSF (yeast-derived)	Leukine	Autologous BMT engraftment or failure	Immunex	Market
GM-CSF (yeast-derived)	Leukine	Neutropenia induced by chemo. In AML	Immunex	Market
GM-CSF (yeast-derived)	Leukine	Allogeneic BMT engraftment or failure	Immunex	Market
GM-CSF (yeast-derived)	Leukine	Mobilization of autologous PBPCs post-chemo.	Immunex	Market
GM-CSF (liquid formulation)	Leukine	BMT engraftment or failure	Immunex	Market
GM-CSF (yeast-derived)	Leukine	Reduce infections in neonatal sepsis	Immunex	Phase III*
GM-CSF (yeast-derived)	Leukine	Trauma	Immunex	Phase II
GM-CSF (yeast-derived)	Leukine	Treat fungal infections in AIDS patients resistant to fluconazole	Immunex	Phase II
Stem cell factor	Stemogen	Hematopoietic disorders	Amgen	Phase II/III

Appendix 2. Myeloid Growth Factors.

Product Description	Trade Name	Indication	Company (Partner)	Status
Interferon alpha-2a	Roferon A	AIDS-related Kaposi's sarcome	Genentech (Hoffmann-LaRoche)	Market
Interferon alpha-2a	Roferon A	Hairy cell leukemia	Genentech (Hoffmann-LaRoche)	Market
Interferon gamma-1b	Actimmune	Chronic granulomatous disease	Genentech	Market
Consensus interferon	Infergen	Hepatitis C treatment	Amgen	Market
Interferon alpha-2b	Intron A	Gential warts	Biogen (Schering-Plough)	Market
Interferon alpha-2b	Intron A	Hepatitis C treatment	Biogen (Schering-Plough)	Market
Interferon alpha-2b	Intron A	Hepatitis B treatment	Biogen (Schering-Plough)	Market
Interferon beta-1a	Avonex	Hepatitis B, hepatitis C	Biogen	Phase II
Interferon beta-1a	Avonex	Genital warts	Biogen (Schering-Plough)	Phase II
Interferon alpha-2b w/AZT	—	HIV/AIDS	Biogen (Schering-Plough)	Phase II
Interferon alpha-2b w/ddl	—	HIV/AIDS	Biogen (Schering-Plough)	Phase II
PEG-interferon alpha-2b	PEG-Intron A	Hepatitis	Enzon (Shering Corp.)	Phase I
Interferon-alpha-n3	ALFERON n	Refractory or recurring external genital warts in adults	Interferon Sciences	Market
Interferon-alpha-n3	Alferon-N	HIV/AIDS	Interferon Sciences	Phase III
Interferon-alpha-n3	Alferon-N	Chronic hepatitis C	Interferon Sciences	Phase III
Low dose oral formulation of interferon-alpha-n3	Alferon-N	HIV/AIDS	Interferon Sciences	Phase III

Appendix 3. Interferons.

Product Description	Trade Name	Indication	Company (Partner)	Status
TGF-Beta-2	–	Dermal ulcers	Celtrix (Genzyme Tissue repair)	Phase I/II
TGF-Beta-2	–	Multiple sclerosis	Celtrix (Genzyme Tissue Repair)	Phase I
TGF-Beta-2	–	Multiple sclerosis	Genzyme Tissue Repair	
TGF-Beta 2	–	Chronic skin ulcers	Genzyme Tissue repair	
TGF-Beta 3	–	Chronic skin wounds	Oncogen Science (Ciba Geigy)	
Lexipafant (PAF antagonist – IV)	–	Pancreatitus (acute)	British Biotech	Phase. III
Lexipafant (PAF antagonist – oral)	–	Multiple sclerosis	British Biotech	Phase II

Appendix 4. Miscellaneous Biological Products.

Product Description	Trade Name	Indication	Company (Partner)	Status
BAY-X-1351		Septic shock	Celltech (Bayer))	Phase III
CDP 571 (BAY10-3356)		Autoimmune disease	Celltech (Bayer)	Phase II
CMB 401 (CDP671-anti-PEM Ab)		Ovarian Cancer	Celltech (AHP)	Phase IIa
CMA 676 (CDP 771-anti-CD33 Ab)		Acute myeloid leukemia	Celltech (AHP)	Phase I/II
CDP 850 (anti-E-selectin Ab)		Psoriasis	Celltech	Phase I/II
CDP 835 (SCH5700-anti-IL5 Ab)		Asthma	Celltech (Schering Plough)	Preclinical
CDP 855 (anti-class II MHC)		Multiple sclerosis	Celltech	Preclinical
Anti-T cell Ab		Transplant rejection	Celltech	Preclinical
GPIIb/IIIa inhibitor (c7E3 Fab)	Reo-Pro®	Inhibit platelet aggregation in angioplasty	Eli Lilly (Centocor)	Market 12/94
Anti-tumor MAb (17-1A)	Panorex®	Colorectal cancer	Glaxo-Wellcome (Centocor)	Phase III
Mouse MAb fragment to myosin	Myoscint®	Cardiac imaging agent-MI	Centocor	Approved 7/96
HA1A	Centoxin®	Fulminant meningococcemia	Eli Lilly (Centocor)	Phase III
Mouse MAb fragment to fibrin	Fibriscint®	Blood clot imaging agent	Centocor	Phase III
AntiTNF chimeric MAb (c2)	CenTNF™	Autoimmune disease	Centocor	Phase II
Anti-CD4 MAb (CMT 412)	Centara	T cell lymphoma and rheumatoid arthritis	Centocor	Phase I/II
MAb to Factor VIIa (12D10)	Corsevin M	Adjunct in angioplasty	Centocor (Corvas)	Phase I/II
Indium-111 labelled Ab	OncoScint®	Tumor imaging	Cytogen	Market 12/92
Yttrium-90 labelled Ab	OncoRad®	Treatment of prostate cancer	Cytogen	Phase II
Anti-HER2 humanized MAb	Herceptin™	Breast cancer	Genentech	Phase III
IDEC-C2B8	Rituxan™	Relapse low grade NHL	IDEC (Genentech)	Marketed 1998
Primatized CE9.1 (antiCD4Abs)		Severe asthma	IDEC (SKB)	Phase II
IDEC-In 2B8 (Yttrium-conjugaed Pan B Ab)		Non-Hodgkin's lymphoma	IDEC (Genentech)	Phase II
105AD7 (Anti-idiotype Ab targeting gp 72)		Colorectal cancer vaccine	ImClone	Phase II

Appendix 5. Antibodies.

Product Description	Trade Name	Indication	Company (Partner)	Status
BEC-2 (Antiidiotype AB targeting GD3)		Malignant melanoma	ImClone	Phase II
C225 (anti-EGF receptor mouse MAB)		Advance head & neck cancer	ImClone	Phase II
Anti-B4-bR (Blocked ricin)	Oncolysin® B	B cell non-Hodgkin's lymphoma	ImmunoGen	Phase III
CMV Immunoglobulin	CytoGam®	CMV reduction in kidney transplants	Medimmune	Market 4/90
RSV immunoglobulin	RespiGam®	RSV disease prevention	Medimmune	Market 1/96
Medi-500 (T10B9) anti-T cell MAb		Prevention of graft versus host disease in BMT patients	Medimmune	Phase III
Medi 493 (humanized RSV MAb)		Prevention of RSV disease	Medimmune	Phase III
BTI-322 (anti-CD2 MAb)		Organ rejection	Medimmune	Phase II
Medi-491 B19 parovirus vaccine		B19 parovirus infection	Medimmune	Phase I
Medi-490 rBCG Lyme disease vaccine		Lyme disease prevention	Medimmune	Phase I
Anti-digoxin Fab	Digibind	Digoxin overdose	Glaxo-Wellcome	Marketed
Human Immunoglobuline	Gammagard, Gamimune-N, Gammar-P	Thrombocytopenia, immunodeficiency	Baxter, Bayer, Amour	Marketed
Anti-hepatitis B immunoglobulin	HBIG	Prevention of hepatitis B	Bayer	Marketed
Anti-CD3 MAb or OKT3	Muramab	Prevention of graft rejection	Orthro biotech	Marketed
Antithymocyte immunoglobulin	ATGAM	Prevention of acute graft rejection	Upjohn-Pharmaciae	Marketed
Anti-RH factor	RhoGam	RH factor incompatibility Gamulin Rh+		Marketed

Appendix 5. Continued.

153

Index